Joseph S Green    Piet G de Boer

# AO Principles of Teaching and Learning

Joseph S Green
Piet G de Boer

# AO Principles of Teaching and Learning

with personal anecdotes

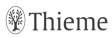

Illustrations: Sandro Isler, nougat gmbh, CH-4056 Basel
Layout and typesetting: AO Publishing, CH-8600 Dübendorf

Library of Congress Cataloging-in-Publication Data is available from the publisher.

Copyright © 2005 by AO Publishing, Switzerland, Clavadelerstrasse, CH-7270 Davos Platz
Distribution by Georg Thieme Verlag, Rüdigerstrasse 14, DE-70469 Stuttgart and
Thieme New York, 333 Seventh Avenue, US-New York, NY 10001

Printed in Switzerland by Kürzi Druck AG, CH-8840 Einsiedeln

ISBN 3-13-141051-5
ISBN 1-58890-365-6

# Contributors

## Editors

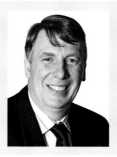

Piet G de Boer, FRCS
AO International
Marlborough House
York Business Park
UK-York, YO26 6RW

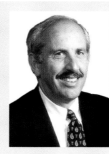

Joseph S Green, PhD
President, Professional Resource
Network, Inc.
Associate Consulting Professor
Duke University School of Medicine
12824 Morehead
US-Chapel Hill, NC 27517

## Authors

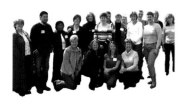

AOUK ORP Speciality Section
Purey Cust Nuffield Hospital
Precentor's Court
UK-York, YO1 7EL

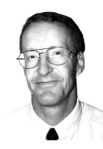

Richard Buckley, MD, FRCSC
Associate Professor
University of Calgary, Surgery
Foothills Medical Center
1403 29 Street NW
CA-Calgary, AB T2N 2T9

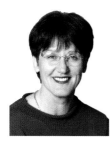

Review ORP
Susanne Bäuerle
AO International
Operating Room Personnel
Clavadelerstrasse
CH-7270 Davos Platz

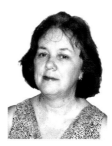

Linda Casebeer, PhD
Associate Director
University of Alabama School of Medicine
Division of CME
1521 11th Ave S
US-Birmingham, AL 35294-4551

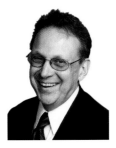

David Davis, MD
Associate Dean
University of Toronto
Faculty of Medicine
Continuing Education Offices
500 University Ave, 6th Floor, Suite 650
CA-Toronto, ON 5G 1V7

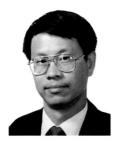

KokSun Khong, MD, FRCSG
Mt. Elizabeth Medical Centre 16-03/04
KS Khong Orthopaedic Practice
3 Mount Elizabeth
SG-Singapore, 228510

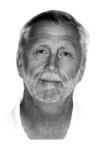

Robert D Fox, EdD Prof.
University of Oklahoma
College of Education
100 McCarter Hall
US-Norman, OK 73072

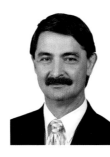

John R Kues, PhD
Assistant Dean of CME
Professor of Family Medicine
University of Cincinnati
PO Box 670567
US-Cincinnati, OH 45267-0567

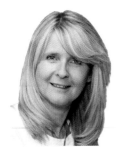

Lisa Hadfield-Law, RGN
Bailey's Consulting
Church Street, Charlbury
UK-Oxfordshire, OX7 3PR

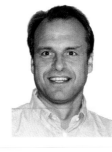

Roger KJ Simmermacher, MD, PhD
University Medical Center Utrecht
Department of Surgery
PO Box 85500
NL-3508 GA Utrecht

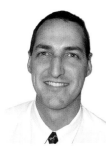

Ian Harris, MD
Liverpool Hospital
Orthopaedic Department
Level 1, Clinical Building
AU-Liverpool NSW 2170

# Foreword

Why does the AO offer such a book? When the AO was founded 45 years ago, one of the principles was to provide education to surgeons in the use of the revolutionary techniques of open reduction and internal fixation of fractures (ORIF). The attractive and numbered sets of AO instruments and implants could only be acquired, if a surgeon had attended a 5-day AO course with hands-on workshops in Davos, Switzerland. The lecturers and table instructors for the practical exercises were the AO founding members themselves. Some were better teachers than others, but instructing junior surgeons was not new to them as this is part of a surgeon's daily practice in the operating room. As the demand for AO courses rapidly increased and expanded outside Switzerland, the number of faculty members also rose steadily and is growing still. Today, close to 170 AO courses are offered annually worldwide with more than 13,000 surgeons and around 70 ORP courses with over 4,000 operating room personnel of different levels and specialities being instructed in the use of AO techniques.

Today, there are around 3,000 faculty members worldwide who provide high-level education for their younger colleagues. It is clear that it has become increasingly difficult to maintain a high standard of teaching and for that reason AO has involved professional educators to ensure that attention is given to the way AO education is delivered. AO also ensures that the content and messages of the AO philosophy are the core of each course thereby guaranteeing that the original "unité de doctrine" is maintained.

The idea for this book on "AO Principles of Teaching and Learning", which is part of the AO faculty development program, came from Joseph S Green, PhD. The content results from several educators' seminars and tips-for-trainer courses in Davos and in the UK. Every chapter addresses one of the roles an AO faculty member may be assigned to in a course; for example, table instructor, lecturer, moderator of a workshop or discussion group, or course chairman. Each chapter was authored by a team of an experienced senior AO surgeon/AO faculty member and a professional educator. It provides essential information and useful advice on how to perform the different tasks during an AO course. The experience of the AO faculty member is given a theoretical basis by the professional educator. A special chapter is dedicated to the unique challenges of ORP education. The authors have provided a clear and easy-to-read text with many useful hints on how to improve the performance of surgeons as teachers.

The book focuses on teaching and learning within AO courses. It may, however, also be of interest for other groups involved in adult education. The AO concept of blended learning with lectures, workshops, discussion groups, as well as on- and off-line distance learning is a model that could be usefully followed by many others in the field of medical education.

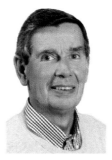

Thomas P Rüedi, MD, FACS
Davos, September 2004

# Table of contents

Authors   Piet G de Boer, Joseph S Green

# 1    AO education—introduction

## 1    History

Education has been one of the most important aspects of the AO organization since its formation in 1958. The founders of AO recognized that they would be unable to successfully spread their principles and philosophy throughout the world unless they actively became involved in the education of their peers. AO courses commenced in Davos in 1960 and from the very first course, practical, hands-on skill training was an integral part of the AO educational endeavor.

The AO pioneers also understood that patient care could be enhanced if education were offered not only to practicing surgeons but also to those ORP (operating room personnel) colleagues who assisted them in their operations. Hence, ORP education and surgeons' education were linked in the earliest days of AO.

Early AO courses had two elements—lectures and practicals. Lectures were traditionally given with dual 35 mm projection and had a relatively standard format. This consisted of an introduction followed by principles of the topic, copious clinical illustrations, and some results relating to the topic under discussion. Practicals were initially carried out using cadaveric bone and the instruments and implants needed for the surgery in real life. Plastic bones were introduced in the early 1970s. Videos were produced at an early stage to enhance the learning experience and table instructors were used to supervise the activities of the course participants. The characteristic way in which an AO practical ran was for the practical director to run the video in its entirety and then allow the participants to proceed with the practical under the critical gaze of their table instructors.

AO teaching was spectacularly successful from its inception. The use of real instrumentation and implants and the use of plastic bone models were truly innovative in the educational field. The setting of the course in Davos was also an important part of the success of these early courses combining, as it did, the unique ambience of a Swiss ski resort in winter with access to the intellectual and research base of the organization. This educational format was successfully exported throughout the world and found widespread acceptance in many countries.

In the early 1990s it became clear that the educational value of the courses might be improved, not so much by changing what was taught, as by changing the way in which education was delivered. David Pitts, PhD, a full-time professional educator was employed by the then President of AO International, Peter Matter, with a remit to try to improve the process of teaching delivered by AO on a worldwide basis. David Pitts worked closely with David Rowley, Professor of Orthopaedic Surgery at Dundee University, Scotland. David organized very successful educational seminars in Davos in the 1990s which resulted in widespread acceptance amongst those members present that improving the way in which we taught would significantly improve the learning outcomes for the course participants. In 1997 William M Murphy, FRCSI, Epsom, United Kingdom, James F Kellam, MD, North Carolina, USA, and Joe Schatzker, MD, Toronto, Canada, combined to produce the modular principles course, the first AO course which had a written syllabus and defined learning outcomes. The development of the principles course and the acceptance that teaching techniques were important began the second revolution in AO teaching. This book is designed to take that process one stage further.

## 2    Organization of the book

This book has been written to be used by existing and future AO faculty in order to enhance their skills in the many educational roles they play within AO and in their own practice setting. It is essentially a handbook on how to maximize the educational success of each AO course.

The book is divided into chapters, each relating to a specific role within an AO course:

Chapter 2—How to be a course chairman
Chapter 3—How to run a discussion group
Chapter 4—How to run a practical
Chapter 5—How to be a table instructor
Chapter 6—How to give a lecture

Each chapter outlines the duties and responsibilities of the faculty member in each of the roles. Each chapter is divided into those tasks which must be completed before the course begins, those tasks which are to be undertaken during the precourse, those tasks which are to be undertaken during the course and, finally, what things need to be done after the course. Each chapter is written jointly by an experienced AO clinical educator and a professionally trained expert in educational research, theory, and practice. Each chapter aims, not only to give practical advice to those faculty members undertaking a particular role, but also to give those faculty members the theoretical rationale for the educational advice that is given. References are provided within each chapter to allow each individual to better understand the theo-

retical basis for the practice that is being advocated. The book is primarily to be used as a pragmatic handbook and not as an academic reference book for educational theory. It is hoped that reading a specific chapter will become standard practice before AO faculty undertake a given educational assignment within AO.

A separate chapter—7 How to run an ORP course—is included to discuss the particular needs of ORP education within the existing AO course structure. Faculty teaching on ORP courses will need to read, not only this chapter, but also the chapter that relates to the individual tasks that they have been asked to perform within the course. ORP education, which has always been a keystone of AO educational activity, has many common points with physician education. However, there are also issues, particularly with regard to culture and gender, which give rise to unique challenges for ORP education throughout the world.

The book concludes with chapter 8—a summary of the most important principles presented in the chapters and a look forward to the future with a discussion of five key development areas within AO education: self-assessment, practice-based learning, educational technology, quality improvement, and knowledge management tools.

Two very important educational subjects are relevant to several of the chapters—audience response system (ARS) and evaluation. These will be discussed in this introductory chapter and are mentioned again within some sections of the remaining text.

## 3    Audience response system (ARS)

These systems are usually referred to as ARS and have been in existence for many years. ARS technology was developed to engage learners in the learning process during lectures by eliciting their responses to questions developed by the expert faculty. Until the 1990s ARS was a very expensive tool that was hard wired into a specific conference room or lecture hall. More recently, wireless electronic connections have developed and ARS has become mobile. These systems can be set up in any room and can be shipped all over the world. They have, therefore, become much more popular. The key advancement offered by these systems is that they allow for learner involvement in the education process. The theory of adult learning has shown that a passive educational setting, such as a lecture, does not facilitate learner involvement in the education process. Learners in lectures are less likely to actually learn what is being taught, less likely to retain what they might have learned, and certainly less likely to apply what they have learned in their practice setting. As one ancient Chinese proverb states, "Tell me and I shall forget, show me and I may remember, involve me and I will understand…". In more recent times, the renown educator John Dewey in his landmark book in 1938 entitled the *Theory of Inquiry* wrote: "He has to see on his own behalf…the relation between means and methods employed and results achieved…nobody else can see for him and he can't see just by being told…".

■ ⅲ    **Involvement of the course participants is now an integral part of the AO educational philosophy and is the reason why we stress the use of small groups, hands-on practical experiences, and, more recently, the use of ARS to enhance the lecture learning experience.**

The audience response system offers quick tabulations of audience responses for:

- Discussion.
- Speaker control of when and how responses are displayed.
- The addition of impromptu questions during the session.
- The ability to continue the session in an unplanned direction with participants.
- Participant anonymity.

In addition, an ARS enables the lecturer to immediately obtain a more detailed assessment of participant demographics (to tailor the case presentation and discussion appropriately) and to gather evaluation data.

How can ARS be used to facilitate learning, retention, and application to practice? There are several appropriate uses of this technology including: pre-post test of knowledge, pre-post attitude inventories, learner profiles, case studies, inserted questions, and comparison data.

## Pre-post test of knowledge

The first use is for pre-post test of knowledge and the relevant question to ask is "What do the learners know?" In order to use the ARS effectively, the following suggestions need to be taken into consideration:

- Select most important concepts to be learned.
- Provide immediate feedback to learners.
- Assure results are known only by learners.
- Allow learners to compare results with peers.
- Test for application of knowledge in real world setting.
- Use same test items for post test (or pick from same pool of questions).
- Use multiple-choice questions to assure learner can make fine discriminations.

If the intent is to use the ARS for testing purposes, a few principles about building test items are provided:

- Test items should relate to important content objectives.
- Should be based on application of knowledge, not memorization of facts.
- Use multiple choice whenever possible; true-false questions are too easy to guess correctly.
- Keep correct answer from being the longest.
- Spread correct answer around among ABCD alternatives.
- Avoid double negative answers.
- Base possible wrong answers on real-world mistakes.
- Avoid "all of the above" or "none of the above"; if used, make it the correct answer sometimes and the incorrect answer other times.
- Make sure all answers flow grammatically from the stem.

All of these suggestions should be helpful to answer the question of: "Are you testing what is important?"

## Pre-post attitude inventory

The second use is for pre-post attitude inventory and the relevant question is "What do the learners feel?" For this use the following suggestions are made:

- Identify attitudes critical to learning material or skills.
- Use 5-point Likert scales.
- Provide feedback to learners of typical (average) response.
- Show changes at completion of activity to reinforce learning.

## Learner profiles

The third use is for learner profiles and the relevant question is "Who are the learners?" The suggestions for this use include:

- Identify important demographics such as age, sex, years since residency, specialty.
- Determine primary motivator for attending (eg, content, location, credit, faculty, sponsor).
- Assess primary learning needs before and after activity.
- Remain flexible—adapt to the identified needs.

## Case studies

The fourth use is for case studies and the relevant question is "Can learners apply what they have learned?" Suggestions for this use include:

- Link case(s) to major learning objectives, not obscure facts.
- Use one long case throughout activity.
- Use multiple cases within the activity.
- Require learners to answer application of knowledge questions about case(s), not memorization questions about facts.
- Remain flexible on future content depending on learner answers.

## Inserted questions

The fifth use is for inserted questions and the relevant question is "Are learners focused and do they already know this?"

Suggestions for this use include:

- Relate questions to major learning objectives.
- Use questions when knowledge is critical to proceeding with new content.
- Provide immediate feedback to learners so they learn what they don't know.
- Insert at random times to keep attention of learners.

## Comparison data

The sixth and final use that will be described is for comparison data to answer the question "How can you help learners know where they stand?"

Suggestions for this use include:

- Compare current learner performance to past participants.
- Contrast current learner performance to local, regional, or national data.
- Provide learner with pre-post learning data.
- Compare current learner performance with average of peers.

As you can see, if you are offered the opportunity to use the ARS, you have a number of options. However, some careful planning is required. The ARS poll is usually projected on another screen and is controlled through another computer with the appropriate software. It is necessary for the speaker or moderator to submit ARS questions on a page of the PowerPoint presentation beforehand. These questions are identified and duplicated on the ARS computer. When the page is projected by the lecturer, the ARS presenter also projects the same questions and the audience is asked to key in their choice on the keypad. A countdown timer is useful to speed up response. Bar charts show the response and the lecturer and moderator can then comment on the outcome **(Fig 1-1)**.

■ ▥    **ARS sample**

**Your option for definitively treating a displaced femoral midshaft fracture in an adult is:**

A  **Traction by skeletal pin of 20 kg in a Thomas' splint.**

B  **Open reduction and rigid plating with an 8-hole LC-DCP.**

C  **Closed reduction and plating with a 12-hole submuscular LCP.**

D  **Locked unreamed solid intramedullary nail.**

E  **Locked reamed cannulated intramedullary nail.**

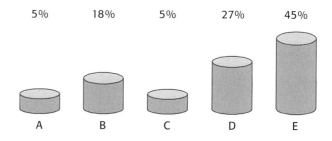

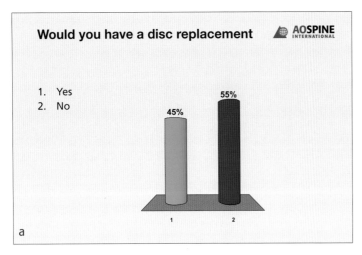
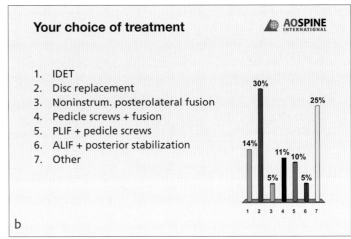

Fig 1-1a–b    Examples of the use of ARS in an AOSpine evidence-based spine surgery seminar in Porto 2004.

In deciding whether a specific AO course should attempt to use ARS technology, it is helpful to look at both those realities that are barriers to its successful use, and those that are facilitators of effective use.

Some of the barriers include: faculty inexperience with ARS, overuse of a good thing, inappropriate questions, lack of flexibility with answers, too many questions, cost of the process, faculty can't use typical presentation, and no one technically qualified to assist faculty. Also, lecturers must remember to allow sufficient time for ARS during their presentations. A typical ARS question, including short discusion of results, will take 2 minutes out of a lecture. Hence it follows that if two ARS questions are to be used during a 15-minute presentation, then that presentation will need to be reduced to 11 minutes in length.

On the other hand, there are also many things that will facilitate effective ARS use: faculty development, staff training, helpful hints for faculty use, integration with content, PowerPoint presentations, use of educational consultant, and available financial support. Because of the complexity of creating successful ARS material, banks of appropriate questions are being created by various national AO bodies, most notably AO North America.

AO International has purchased an ARS system which can be made available for any course worldwide providing sufficient notice is given.

## 4    Evaluation

In a recent effort to update the AO course evaluation system and processes a question was asked of those in charge—how useful is the information you have been gathering in your course evaluations? The answer was that most of the information that was being gathered was neither surprising nor particularly helpful in improving the courses. Each course had a specific evaluation instrument that was handed out to each participant. The evaluation form focused primarily on the quality of the faculty, along with other educational and logistical processes. Participants had to keep the rather lengthy form with them all week and remember to provide feedback on each faculty person after each session—a burdensome job. When you calculate the number of separate courses over a 2-week period and the number of participants in each course you can begin to understand the enormity of the data summary task that faced this AO staff each year after the meeting was over. This information was summarized and given to the appropriate course chairman in preparation for the next year's events. In addition, those in charge were not convinced that the courses were actually improving as a result of this monumental effort. The goal of this review was to try to create a process that was more efficient, but also more effective in enhancing the quality of the courses in a demonstrable way.

What was created in the fall of 2003 was a new process to be piloted during the Davos courses in December of that year. The process was based on a few very important adult educational principles:

- Linking new knowledge to previous experience.
- Having a clear vision of what should be achieved.
- Desiring involvement in the learning process.
- Seeking reinforcement of what has been learned [1, 2, 3].

**Who was involved?**
Rather than involving everyone in each course, the new plan called for each course to be assigned two expert faculty "course evaluators". Their job was to work with a small focus group of about 8–10 randomly selected participants to evaluate various aspects of their course. These two faculty members were briefed about the process the first morning of the course and told about their primary functions—gather data from the focus group members about their expectations and perceptions and compare and contrast those with their own views as expert faculty. The two faculty members then summarized and analyzed the data in order to render a practical, useful set of suggested improvements for the course to the course chairman who then finalized a report for their course to the AO Education Board and to the next course chairman.

**What was the focus?**
Although the performance of the faculty was still an important element of the course evaluation process, there were a number of additional areas that were scrutinized:

- Meeting of course objectives.
- Appropriateness of the content for the specific objectives.

- Effectiveness of the faculty in involving the learners in the learning experience.
- Effectiveness of the hands-on/practical instructors.
- Helpfulness of the course materials (videos, bones, soft tissues/foam models), and equipment.
- Adequacy of the time required to learn a particular skill.
- Adequacy of the feedback on their performance.
- Helpfulness of case studies.
- Effectiveness of educational formats (lectures, discussion groups, fire-side discussions, audience response system, workshops, etc).
- Scientific rigor and objectivity of the content.
- Ability to apply what has been learned back in the practice setting.
- Effectiveness of the logistical support.
- Suggested enhancements for the course.

**When did these evaluations occur?**
For each course, the faculty experts met with their focus group before the activity started, in the middle of the sessions, and after the course ended in order to determine a range of views on various aspects of the quality of the course. For instance, at the first meeting the focus group was asked whether they had been sent precourse material and if they had read the course objectives. At the focus group in the middle of the course, more time was spent evaluating changes that could be made immediately to improve the quality of the activity. At the final meeting, the participants were asked about such things as changes they planned to make in their practice. During the spring of 2004 a follow-up questionnaire was sent to a sampling of participants. This instrument dealt with what they have actually accomplished as a result of the course. The alternative responses included:

- Did not learn anything new.
- Re-confirmed that what I was doing was appropriate.
- Learned something new, but did not want to use it in my practice.
- Learned something new, want to use it in my practice, but have not been able to do so.
- Learned something new and have used it in my practice.

The participants were asked to assess each of the course objectives against the above possible outcomes. They were also asked to explain why they were not able to use what they had learned (which, hopefully suggested new, necessary content for the next year). In addition, feedback was solicited about additional content needed, most valuable aspects of the course in Davos, and any additional ideas for improvement.

**Next steps**
Preliminary findings have already been given to the course chairmen. These reports are full of wonderful suggestions for improvements in all aspects of each of the courses. The overall evaluation process will be fine tuned for next December's courses with the suggestions that several of the faculty experts and participants have already made to AO.

## 5    Bibliography

1. **Bennett NL, Davis DA, Green JS, et al** (2000) Continuing medical education: a new vision of the professional development of physicians. *Acad Med*; 75:1167–1172.
2. **Barnes BE** (1999) Evaluation of learning in health care organizations. *J Contin Educ Health Prof*; 19:227–233.
3. **Davis DA, Barnes BE, Fox RD** (2003) *The Continuing Professional Development of Physicians: From Research to Practice.* Chicago: AMA Press.

### Suggestions for further reading

- **Abrahamson S, Baron J, Elstein AS, et al** (1999) Continuing medical education for life: eight principles. *Acad Med*; 74(12):1288–1294.
- **Amin Z** (2000) Theory and practice in continuing medical education. *Ann Acad Med Singapore*; 29(4):498–502.
- **Bennett NL, Davis DA, Easterling WE Jr, et al** (2000) Continuing medical education: a new vision of the professional development of physicians. *Acad Med*; 75(12):1167–1172.
- **Brandt BL** (1996) Cognitive Learning Theory and Continuing Health Professions Education. *J Contin Educ Health Prof*; 16:197–202.
- **Davis DA, O'Brien MA, Freemantle N, et al** (1999) Impact of formal continuing medical education: do conferences, workshops, rounds, and other traditional continuing education activities change physician behavior or health care outcomes? *JAMA*; 282:867–874.
- **Ebell MH, Shaughnessy A** (2003) Information mastery: integrating continuing medical education with the information needs of clinicians. *J Contin Educ Health Prof*; 23(Suppl 1):53–62.
- **Freemantle N, Harvey EL, Wolf F, et al** (2000) Printed educational materials: effects on professional practice and health care outcomes. *Cochrane Database Syst Rev*; (2):CD000172.
- **Hunt DL, Haynes RB, Hanna SE, et al** (1998) Effects of computer-based clinical decision support systems on physician performance and patient outcomes: a systematic review. *JAMA*; 280(15):1339–1346. Comment in: *ACP J Club* (1999) 130(3):79. *JAMA* (1998) 280(15):1360–1361.
- **Leist JC, Green JS** (2000) Congress 2000: a continuing medical education summit with implications for the future. *J Contin Educ Health Prof*; 20(4):247–251.
- **Mamary EM, Charles P** (2000) On-site to on-line: barriers to the use of computers for continuing education. *J Contin Educ Health Prof*; 20(3):171–175.
- **Manning PR, DeBakey L** (2001) Continuing medical education: the paradigm is changing. *J Contin Educ Health Prof*; 21(1):46–54.
- **Markert RJ, O'Neill SC, Bhatia SC** (2003) Using a quasi-experimental research design to assess knowledge in continuing medical education programs. *J Contin Educ Health Prof*; 23(3):157–161.
- **Robertson MK, Umble KE, Cervero RM** (2003) Impact studies in continuing education for health professions: update. *J Contin Educ Health Prof*; 23(3):146–156.

Authors   Richard Buckley, Joseph S Green

# 2   How to be a course chairman

## 1   Introduction

Becoming an AO course chairman for a CME (continuing medical education) activity targeted at enhancing the clinical knowledge and skills of colleagues is an important educational responsibility for a physician. The chairman must understand how to serve this function in an effective and efficient manner. The course chairman must become knowledgeable about and competent in multiple arenas such as:

- Identifying learning needs.
- Making planning decisions about educational formats, methods, and media.
- Creating content that satisfies identified learning outcomes.
- Selecting quality faculty.
- Helping course participants to translate new information back to their practice setting.
- Managing resources and time.
- Serving as a master motivator.
- Measuring outcomes.

"Among the conditions that contribute to the ability of an educational activity to create an impact, two are predominant. First, the activity must be based on something the course participant has the need and motivation to learn; second, the activity must be designed to present what the course participant needs to know in a manner that will promote learning" [1].

## 1.1   Objectives

This chapter is designed to help AO course chairmen. Much of what is written about in this chapter reflects an organizational algorithm and style that has been developed over time by the volunteer AO educators to provide useful guidelines for this difficult task. In addition, the lessons learned from the literature about how to successfully plan continuing medical education activities for physicians will also be shared with the reader to enhance their perspective about this educational responsibility. Course chairmen must be deliberate and organized in their approach to this complicated responsibility, requiring involvement of many people from many different geographical locations with very different educational planning and teaching styles.

- ■  ▦  **It is the goal of the authors that by the end of this chapter, the reader should be able to:**

  - ▦  **Organize an effective AO course.**
  - ▦  **Understand important steps in the educational process for facilitating the learning of colleagues.**
  - ▦  **Use available faculty and other resources in the most effective way for course delivery.**
  - ▦  **Manage their planning time effectively and provide timely motivation to all those involved in the process.**
  - ▦  **Consider how to avoid or manage problems that might arise during the planning or implementation of a course.**
  - ▦  **Evaluate the degree to which goals and objectives for the course were or were not reached.**

## 1.2 Tasks of the course chairman

To allow effective delivery of a successful course, the job description of the course chairman includes the following tasks:

- Provide leadership to administrative staff and course teachers.
- Motivate participants to want to learn.
- Provide a course that uses the best possible educational strategies based on identified learning needs.
- Decide upon appropriate teaching styles and learning techniques for the most effective dissemination of knowledge.
- Deliver a course that will stimulate participants to return home with the knowledge, skills, and attitudes necessary to practice continuous quality improvement in patient care and deliver high-quality and cost-sensitive patient outcomes.

■ ▦ **…leadership…motivator…appropriate teaching styles…stimulate participants…**

Being a course chairman is both an honor and a great deal of work. Individuals should accept this task only if they are able to spend the necessary time needed to successfully meet the responsibilities listed above. Most course chairmen have been closely connected to other AO educational roles and have proven to be dedicated, trusted, and able to accomplish the task at hand.

This chapter describes the responsibilities of a course chairman in a way that follows the time frames of chairing an AO course: before the course (very early: 18–12 months; early: 12–6 months); as the course nears (6–3 months); at the precourse; at the course; and, immediately after the course (1 week). We describe course planning as a linear process, but in reality the course chairman is steadily moving forward completing certain tasks before others can be handled, while constantly revisiting and revising other planning decisions.

Recent, definitive work on educational planning suggests that the most effective model is an interactive model of program planning based on seven assumptions [2]:

- Focusing on learning and change.
- Recognizing the nonsequential nature of the planning process.
- Discerning the importance of context and negotiation.
- Attending to preplanning and last-minute changes.
- Honoring and taking into account diversity and cultural differences.
- Accepting that program planners work in different ways.
- Understanding that program planners are course participants.

This model is built on the work of many educational researchers having studied curriculum development processes since 1949. Those who actually do the planning of educational activities often do not use all the steps in a particular model and may not even call one part of the process the same as others do [3]. This chapter proposes a unique planning model based on the experience of AO faculty members.

## 2    Before the course

**Criteria for deciding about whether you could be an effective course chairman:**

- **Are you committed to the AO educational mission?**
- **Do you have the time available to give to this important responsibility?**
- **Are you willing to learn how to improve your skills as a course planner?**
- **Do you work well with different types of colleagues (different specialties, different cultures, various levels of management)?**
- **Are you organized and deliberate enough to accomplish large, complicated tasks?**
- **Have you had some experiences similar to this in the past and enjoyed the process and outcomes?**
- **Do you feel you have many good ideas on how to improve the process?**
- **Are you willing to listen to others' critique of how you perform, learn from that experience, and make your course better than it has been in the past?**
- **Are you willing to ask for help and assistance when you need it?**

The time before the course can be divided into the following phases.

The first phase ideally begins around 18 months prior to an AO activity and lasts about 6 months. The tasks in this phase include: identifying general content and course participants, establishing a planning team and timelines, and finalizing location and budget.

The next set of tasks (about 12–6 months before the actual course) focusses on the details related to the course design, as well as to the administrative and logistical support. What will be described are a series of intertwined decisions that need to be made or managed by the course chairman in collaboration with the other team members. Ideally, the other members of the team have been empowered by the chairman to carry out their planning in a coordinated way. As pointed out by Conner [4], the most effective leaders create a planning environment where those who have useful contributions to the decision making are heard and those who need to make the decisions are open to relevant input. Setting up such an environment is the central role of the chairman.

The types of decisions that will be made include:

- Assessing learners' needs.
- Identifying and inviting appropriate faculty.
- Selecting formats, methods, and media.
- Creating logistical and administrative support systems.
- Evaluating the course.
- Managing the course and avoiding common pitfalls.

Thirdly, there are three responsibilities that the chairman has during this third phase (6–3 months in advance) of course development:

- Completing planning and logistical details.
- Collaborating with other course chairmen if more than one course is being held at the same time.
- Planning the precourse faculty meeting.

### 2.1 Identifying general content and course participants (18–12 months in advance)

Many courses have been in existence for several years. If this is so, your very first step, as a newly appointed course chairman, is to learn everything you can about the last course. Did it succeed in meeting the identified goals and objectives? Reading the course evaluation report—if available—is a useful way to understand the realities of the last course and determine what might need to change this year. Meeting with the past course chairman and/or planning team allows understanding of the context around which this year's planning must be carried out. This discussion should focus on the goals of the upcoming course and any changes that may be necessary. As described by Moon, the agreement about course goals and possible outcomes serves two purposes:

- Identify and communicate the intention of the course planners and teachers.
- Articulate what the course participants will learn and be able to apply back in their practice setting after the course.

As Moon [5] goes on to point out, making the potential changes in the participants' practice explicit will encourage the learners to critically assess their current level of practice and increase the chances of actually making the changes when they leave the course. The second benefit in making the goals and outcomes explicit to the planning team is that it will assist them to make other planning decisions based on what will bring about the desired changes in the course participant.

Techniques in orthopedic and trauma surgery change rapidly over time. In order to decide on general content and target audience, the newly named course chairman must assess recent trends within the surgical environment that must affect course themes. Communication with fellow course chairmen and others in the AO will help to produce any new ideas to be introduced at the course. For AO courses using cadaveric material, AO International set up specific guidelines to be adhered to—see Appendix.

In order to make decisions about who to enroll as course participants, it is important to understand how the various courses fit into surgical training. The AO Principles Course is known to be an entry-level course for surgical trainees who are in their first two years of training. The AO Principles Course runs regularly in many different parts of the world to provide a baseline level of education to surgical trainees. The minimum entry level for enrolling in an AO Advances Course is successful completion of an AO Principles Course. Entry-level criteria for participants in AO courses should be established to ensure participants are placed in the proper course.

### ■ ▥ Identifying course participants according to their level of surgical training is crucial.

These criteria can be the basis for a precourse assessment instrument to ensure that the course has the most appropriate learners. This assessment tool will also allow for the effective delivery of a sufficient number

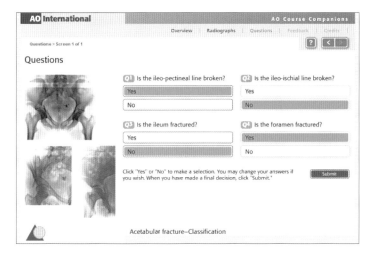

Fig 2-1    Screen shot of an eLearning module for course preassessment.

of courses, given the available administrative staff. The desired end result is the effective functioning of the course with the right physician in the right course at the right time during their training. When multiple skill levels are accepted into a given course, other decisions need to be made to allow for "tracking" of more homogeneous subgroups to deal with application of what was learned to their particular realities. eLearning-based assessment has been successfully used for streaming of course participants at master-level courses (Pohlemann, 2003; **Fig 2-1**).

## 2.2    Establishing a planning team and timelines (18–12 months in advance)

The next step in this process is to build a planning team to assist in carrying out the myriad of tasks that must be accomplished for a successful course. Lundy [6] suggests

that high performing teams are led by decision makers who not only pay attention to content, but also attend to process and principle by establishing open communication systems, encouraging feedback throughout the process, and taking advantage of the different skill sets of other team members. It is also very important to establish careful timelines with course administrative personnel and the co-chairman. Many individuals and groups contribute to a successful course. AO International can provide faculty from around the world. The industrial partner provides logistics' support for the course, local AO groups provide knowledge about the needs of the course participants. There must be a very careful and cooperatively agreed-upon-working strategy for all parties involved. It is useful to have early face-to-face meetings with all the individuals and groups to agree on the content of the course.

Incoming and outgoing course chairmen are excellent resources for course planning. Chairmen are often appointed for 3 years. The first year that a course chairman is involved is a good opportunity to "learn the ropes" of the effective techniques used in a particular course. In the second year the chairman should be responsible for many of the intricate details of the course. By the third year, this chairman should be involved in mentoring their successors. Different chairmen provide different expertise and interests, which may lead to specific assignments or duties. Courses with international chairmen benefit from chairmen's experience gained in courses that take place worldwide.

Finally, it is important to assess the various skill sets that AO members can bring to the planning team. It is very important to include those who can handle administrative duties, meeting planning, logistical support, audiovisual duties, electronic tools such as audience response systems (ARS), and marketing and advertising responsibilities. Whatever skills they bring to the planning process, "each player will contribute more effectively to the extent that they can be helped to become:

- Clearly aware of the group's mission.
- Sensitive to individual differences.
- Willing to listen to others' views.
- Considerate of others' interests and needs.
- Interested in the challenges and opportunities of associates.
- Oriented to long-term progress and success.

The successful team leader will see that existing individual objectives will be compatible with the needs for coordinated overall effectiveness" [6].

### 2.3 Finalizing location and budget (18–12 months in advance)

The establishment of course location and the securing of course resources varies considerably throughout the world. In many areas, education committees take on this role. In other parts of the world this is the responsibility of AO International. The role of the chairman is to assure that the resources made available to produce the course are adequate to meet its goals and that the location selected will facilitate and not hinder the learning that must take place for course participants to reach the desired outcomes. In designing courses for surgeons and other professionals, there are often many approaches that will lead to successful outcomes, some of which are far more expensive than others. The key is to make sure

the decisions made during the planning process take into consideration both effectiveness in meeting objectives and efficiency in not exceeding the budget.

■ ▦ **Initial planning decisions to be made by the course chairman:**

- ▦ **Overall goals of course established.**
- ▦ **Appropriate target audience clarified.**
- ▦ **Team members identified.**
- ▦ **Roles of other course chairmen articulated.**
- ▦ **Course location finalized.**
- ▦ **Budget agreed on.**
- ▦ **Collaboration established with AO staff.**

### 2.4 Assessing course participants' needs (12–6 months in advance)

One of the most important elements of planning for adult health professionals is to obtain information about the participants' expectations so that planners can facilitate decision making about content, faculty, and educational processes. Courses often use precourse needs assessment questionnaires that require course participants to reflect on their knowledge and patient care practices prior to a course [7]. Four sources for gathering needs assessment data on participants are:

- Clinical data bases.
- Chart audit or feedback systems.
- Knowledge or competency assessment.
- Perceived performance.

■ ▥    **The value of understanding course participants' needs:**

▥ **Better equipped to meet course participants' expectations for the course.**
▥ **Assure more relevant outcome objectives and content for course participants.**
▥ **Select most appropriate formats and methods.**
▥ **Select best faculty for specific needs or realities of course participants.**
▥ **Better able to evaluate the degree of need fulfillment.**
▥ **Provide most effective and efficient use of physician course participants' time.**

What are educational needs? For years, educators have described them as the discrepancy between what is and what should be [8]. Today, educators realize that there are both problem-based needs and opportunity-based needs that emanate from an analysis of the relevant healthcare environment of the learners. Problem-based needs result from physicians not practicing at the level required by their specialty; opportunity-based needs, on the other hand, are those that result from the gap between current practice levels and higher possible levels based on new developments, procedures, or technologies entering the marketplace. "The stimulus for engaging in learning often begins when physicians reflect on their practice and engage in learning in order to find a solution to a problem, ensure that skills and abilities are up-to-date, or gain new competencies" [9]. AO provides education on orthopedics and traumatology to surgical trainees and practicing physicians. The needs are usually related to the procedures, technologies, and new products that are an integral part of this surgical environment.

Of the four previously mentioned data sources, the two that seem most appropriate for our courses are the knowledge or competency assessment and perceived performance. AO has not yet developed valuable cognitive or skill-level preassessments for course participants. Course chairmen must, however, think if such an assessment would yield enough valuable data to make the effort worth the time and money that would need to be invested. The result of such an effort would be to ensure that participants are involved in taking the correct course and not involved in a course which is at an inappropriate level, given their training and experience. The need for preassessment becomes greater as the level of the course increases. The AO Principles Courses are suitable for any surgical trainee. Successful participation in an AO Advances Course requires completion of an AO Principles Course and the possession of suitable clinical experience. The problem becomes even more acute at AO Masters Course level.

The chairman's responsibility is to gather enough information about the participants to feel confident that what is being designed as an educational experience will be appropriate for them and will, therefore, lead to an enhancement of their surgical care of patients. If the decision is to gather needs assessment data prior to a course, it should be the minimal amount to give the chairman the confidence that most of the assumptions about the course participants were accurate. This can be done using eLearning-based assessment modules to be completed by the course participants 2 weeks prior to the course. This could also be done by asking a few questions on the course application form, at registration for the course, or during the initial session via an ARS. The types of questions include:

- Demographic information about their level of training and experience.
- Most important new skill desired.
- Amount of experience in what will be taught.
- A case study to determine their typical approach to a common surgical problem to be dealt with in the course.

As a result of these types of surveys, the chairman might be in a position to move someone into a more appropriate course.

■ ▥  **If this strategy is used, course participants must be aware of this possibility before the course begins. The chairman could also change the contents slightly to adjust to the course participants, add a speaker who might be available, or spend more time on certain case studies in the small groups.**

Any or all of these adjustments will only strengthen the course. And, of course, the earlier that these data are available to the planners, the more options they have for improving the course.

## 2.5 Identifying and inviting appropriate faculty (12–6 months in advance)

Identifying and selecting faculty is a critically important function of the course chairman. These decisions are often made more complicated due to geographic considerations related to the audience or attempts to achieve balance within the faculty. Other times, organizational politics "require" the chairman invite a dignitary to join the faculty. The prime criteria, however, ought to be their ability to communicate what they know about the content they have been asked to cover using the format selected. Whether the faculty is asked to give a lecture, lead a discussion group or fire-side chat/discussion, serve as a moderator for a session, provide hands-on skill building in a practical exercise, or evaluate the session, faculty teaching skills are often ignored when faculty is chosen due to the supposed value of the known clinical and research expert. As described by Grosswald [1], it is sometimes much more effective to use a less well-known clinician with outstanding teaching and communication skills, than an expert who can't teach. The role of the chairman is to mix and match individuals selected to serve as faculty to meet all the educational, administrative, and political agendas of the organization in a way that still meets the course outcome objectives.

Enough notice must be given for the invited faculty. A year's notice is probably required for a busy surgeon's schedule. Invited faculty should be dedicated teachers with a mix of interest and experience **(Fig 2-2)**. It is ideal to have gifted teachers who can fill many roles in discussion groups or act as practical directors. In addition, it is

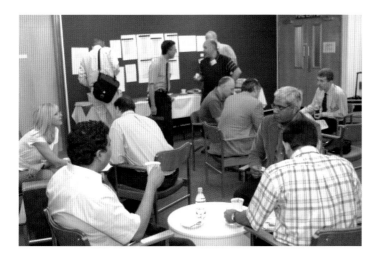

Fig 2-2    Faculty involved in active communication during the course—getting tips and hints for the next session from colleagues as well as educator.

- Be a respected specialist in their subspecialty.
- Facilitate questions from the audience to help them apply what they have learned to the practice setting.
- Use other experts (such as panelists) to clarify questions and issues.
- Involve the audience by asking probing questions or using the ARS.
- Clarify issues related to any potential conflicts of interest by faculty members.
- Keep activity and faculty to agreed upon time-line during presentations.
- Link different presentations together and point out areas of overlap or disagreement to assist the audience in their learning.
- Summarize presentations and provide advance organizers prior to talks to facilitate understanding.
- Use ARS to seek information from learners about current level of knowledge, skills, and attitudes important to the subject matter.
- Willingness to make adjustments in the course, if needed.
- Ability to refrain from using the podium to give their own talk or answer all questions.

very important for future courses that younger teachers are brought along to profit from experienced teachers. First-time table instructors also need sufficient notice to prepare for the course. It is never too early for the course chairman to start the careful assignment of appropriate tasks to faculty, taking into consideration the strengths and weaknesses of each faculty person. For example, certain faculty might make excellent moderators, but less effective table instructors.

Selecting moderators for a course or sections of the course is a very important decision that should be based on whether the physician has the appropriate skills for the task. The skills that a moderator needs (also see 6 How to give a lecture; 3.7.7 Role as a session moderator) to possess are as follows:

As can be seen from this list, the tasks are critical to a successful activity and the decision of who can best accomplish these becomes central to that desired outcome.

■  ▥    **One of the subtle—but important—roles of the chairman is to use individuals in the area where they are most effective and where they can shine the brightest. Sometimes it is much more effective to use a less well-known clinician with outstanding teaching and communication skills, than an expert who can't teach.**

Invitation of faculty must also take into account the individual personalities of surgeons. Certain surgeons have an excellent work ethic in the educational setting and will always be there for the entire course, constantly offering their help. Others are less timely and reliable and may even inexplicably back out of the course at the last moment, providing the course chairman with a serious problem. Regularly communicating with previous and other current course chairmen will help to establish a reliable faculty pool for the successful completion of the course.

## 2.6 Selecting formats, methods, and media (12–6 months in advance)

The classical AO educational format has a long and distinguished history. The newly appointed chairman typically does not make any decisions that change this basic format. What happens within that format is the subject of many decisions that need to be made by the planning team. Usually, the chairman needs to finalize decisions about how to mix and match commonly used educational methods such as:

- Lectures.
- Panel discussions.
- Discussion groups.
- Practical exercises.
- Case-based discussions.
- Videos.
- Web-based information.
- Equipment exhibits.
- Cases provided by faculty.

How these methods are selected and how they are pieced together is a key success factor in meeting the outcome objectives of the course. Caffarella [2] suggests that seven factors need to drive these decisions:

- Background and needs of participants.
- Availability and expertise of faculty.
- Cost.
- Available facilities, technology and equipment.
- Content of activity.
- Desired outcomes.
- Course context.

The ancillary point the author makes is that using several formats accommodates a wide variety of learning styles and approaches to teaching. The role of the course chairman in this process is to assure that the factors listed above are taken into consideration in making the decisions as to what methods will be used and in what order and not just relying on what has been done in the past. **Table 2-1** outlines the features of the most commonly used educational methods that should be considered for AO courses [1].

■ ▥ **AO courses aim to change the practice behavior of the course participants. Certain teaching methods are better than others in bringing this about.**

In order to decide which methods are the most effective, it is first important to understand the process that physicians (and others) go through to change a specific practice behavior. Much of the behavior change literature developed by Prochaska and colleagues [10], who

| Method | Characteristics | Method | Characteristics |
|--------|----------------|--------|----------------|
| Lecture | ▪ Reaches large group.<br>▪ Good for presenting general information of overview.<br>▪ May be effective in changing attitudes.<br>▪ Limited interaction with course participants.<br>▪ Content often forgotten in short periods of time.<br>▪ Effectiveness dependent on presenter. | Observation and practice under supervision | ▪ Provides course participant with a role model.<br>▪ Provides opportunity for practice of skills and for feedback.<br>▪ Course participants can receive experience in real situations.<br>▪ Reaches few course participants at one time.<br>▪ Requires much time. |
| Discussion session | ▪ Actively involves course participants.<br>▪ Enhances understanding and knowledge of course participants.<br>▪ Can be effective in changing attitudes.<br>▪ Better for small group.<br>▪ Requires skilled facilitator. | Reading | ▪ Provides in-depth information.<br>▪ Allows for individual work and pacing.<br>▪ Passive form of learning.<br>▪ May be time-consuming. |
| Panel discussion | ▪ Presents various sides of an issue.<br>▪ May influence attitudes.<br>▪ Limited course participant involvement. | Computer-based instruction | ▪ Involves course participants.<br>▪ Effective for application of learning, practice, and feedback.<br>▪ May be expensive. |
| Demonstration | ▪ Particularly effective in teaching skills or techniques.<br>▪ Allows course participants to see what is expected.<br>▪ Better for small group. | Teleconference | ▪ Reaches course participants at other sites.<br>▪ Relatively inexpensive.<br>▪ Must be well planned. |

Table 2-1   Features of instructional methods.

in 1983 developed a model to describe addictive behavioral change attempts. Their work described five stages of readiness to change:

1. Precontemplation (no need to change identified).
2. Contemplation (change benefits and barriers are considered).
3. Preparation (beginning to plan for change).
4. Action (change happens).
5. Maintenance (of change).

Casebeer and colleagues [11] further describe the difference between expository learning (communication by an expert to a passive learner) to discovery learning (learners involved experientially). Again, if behavioral change is an objective, the more involved the learners are in their own learning, the greater the possibility of change actually happening. Permanent behavioral change is more likely to occur following discussion groups and practicals, than following lectures or panel discussions.

The course chairman will need to understand his role in the orgainzation of practicals, lectures, and discussion groups. (More detailed information and links to the literature will be provided in other chapters within this book: 3 How to run a discussion group; 5 How to be a table instructor; and 6 How to give a lecture.)

### 2.6.1 Practical exercises (practicals)

One of the most successful aspects of AO courses is the practical exercise in which participants have the opportunity to use the equipment and practice specific fracture fixation techniques. The chairman needs to prevent problems by effective advance planning. The first such

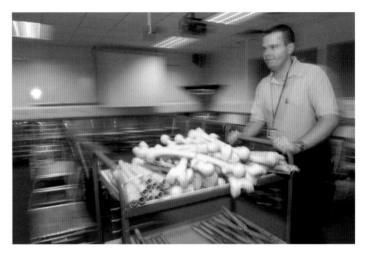

Fig 2-3 Plastic bones, instruments, and implants for practicals—exact planning well in advance is vital to have the necessary material available at the course.

problem is the difficulty in providing enough implants to complete a given practical. Chairmen must communicate with the industrial partner to ensure that implants will be available. Sufficient plastic bones must be supplied (Fig 2-3). Several months may be required for delivery of them depending on participants numbers and the geographic location of the course.

Another effective aspect of a practical exercise involves the careful use of videos. These are produced to reflect the latest gold standard in successfully applying AO techniques. The course chairman must decide (with input from the industrial partner) what practicals will be run at a course to notify the administrative staff in a timely fashion.

■ ▦ **Careful use of teaching videos: Practical exercise videos can become outdated and need to be remade or new implants may require new video production. The course chairman must keep these issues in mind.**

The chairman must set up processes to assure that the appropriate plastic bones to be used by the course participants are available before the course starts. In addition, the faculty member assigned to be the practical director must review the video with enough lead time to make it possible to edit, change or completely redo prior to the course. This matching of video, faculty, and appropriate bone models provide the best opportunity for the participants to have an effective learning experience in the practical.

### 2.6.2   Lectures

Effective lecturers need to be succinct and to-the-point in their delivery of their talks with current, evidence-based information. The presentations should be conceptual and have a logical order and flow. Lecturers need to present their information as general rules, followed by examples of the concepts presented [11]. It is the course chairman's duty to brief those who are selected as lecturers as to the importance of providing content relevant to the outcome objectives and in a manner that has a logical direction and flow for ease of learning on the part of participants. Sufficient time needs to be allocated for the course participants to have their individual questions answered by the faculty. The course chairman can make sure this happens by informing faculty and course participants at the beginning of the course.

The course chairman should also select an effective moderator for each lecture set. They should deliver a seamless approach to the problem that is being presented in a series of lectures. Moderators should coordinate questions and effectively fill gaps in knowledge if desired information is either not presented or not asked in question and answer sessions. The concepts and ideas presented in the lecture need to be reinforced by the moderators to ensure that the participants will be able to implement the concepts in the practical. There is a fine line between being too repetitive and repeating a concept to ensure learning. Making these connections is a critical role played by the course chairman.

Effective use of communication techniques, eg, ARS, enhance course participants' understanding, involvement, and retention. The course chairman, however, must decide to use these electronic tools with enough lead time to make sure they can obtain them and alert the faculty so that they use them. They also need to provide faculty training in the effective use to facilitate learning. When used appropriately, both the audience and the lecturer receive instant feedback to practice-related questions that are posed. When delivered in the context of a lecture, these questions can enhance learning points and principles. It also may allow for each participant to feel involved and more a part of the course and its content.

Other educational methods can be combined with the lecture to enhance participants' interest. These include the presentation of information in debate format, using reaction panels, case studies, and question and answer sessions. On occasion, the use of a roving microphone may bring out more questions from the course participants. The participants in the audience who are too shy to ask a question in a large course may be more comfortable when presented with a question card that can anonymously be taken to the podium for large group discussion. Finally, the course chairman can plan several lectures around different themes or participant-identified, practice-based problems or issues identified through the precourse surveys or cognitive tests.

### 2.6.3 Effective discussion groups

Another form of discovery learning is the small group discussion. These discussion groups should be positioned in the course program to allow the course participants to process what has been given to them in the lecture and practical portions of the course. To assure an effective small group session, the course chairman has to make sure that facilitators (effective discussion leaders) are selected and trained prior to the course. These sessions should include a high level of interaction between the faculty and the participants around interesting cases, practice-based problems, or concerns relevant to the content previously discussed in lectures or practicals. Discussion groups should have no more than 12 participants. With this small number of participants, everyone in the group can participate, and learning will be maximized.

■ ▪ **The right mix or percentage of time that should be spent in these different learning formats—lectures, practicals, discussion groups—is one of the very important design decisions made by the course chairman and planning team.**

These multiple formats, if used appropriately, can assist course participants with different learning style preferences. They can also enhance an individual faculty person's strengths and minimize any of their weaknesses in these important processes of information dissemination and enhancement of surgical skills.

### 2.7 Creating logistic and administrative support systems (12–6 months in advance)

One of the most critical steps in the entire planning process is to establish a productive relationship with the administrative members of the planning team. These members of the planning team help to create a smooth running course that everyone expects as participant or faculty. By setting up a very careful liaison with the important members of the administrative staff for the course, the course chairman will be able to work much more effectively in managing all the planning efforts. In North America, the chairman needs to understand how to use the electronic chat rooms for coordinating communication among all the players. The course chairman also needs to make sure that everyone is using the system. If all are involved and committed to using this paperless technology, the coordination of all aspects of the course is much easier and more efficient. The use of electronic chat rooms will increase in other parts of the world in the future.

### 2.8 Evaluating the course (12–6 months in advance)

Establishing a logical evaluation plan for courses is essential. The course chairman needs to work with the administrative team members to make critical decisions about what will be evaluated, by whom, and how. These decisions need to be based on the information needs of the planning team.

■ ▪ **Evaluation of the course is essential: One common mistake is to continue to use evaluation instruments from the past, regardless of whether they are yielding useful data to the planning process. If the course chairman fails to read the data from the previous years' evaluations, the planning team may be faced with reliving the same problems that had occurred in past courses.**

These data need to help drive decisions about required changes in the current course based on the opinion of past participants. The course chairman must decide what approaches will most likely yield the most useful data. Methods such as focus groups, written participant evaluations, and evaluations from course evaluators are very helpful in establishing the validity of the current course and possible new directions for future courses. There are also other evaluation issues that need to be dealt with by the course chairman. These include:

- Possible use of the ARS for obtaining real-time participant opinions.
- Sampling learners, rather than asking everyone everything.
- Use of scanners to save data analysis time and effort.
- Selection of expert course evaluators.
- Commitment to gathering long-term follow-up data from participants.
- Making ultimate judgments about the value of the course and passing that on to the next chair to assure continuous improvement.

The course chairman must be of the opinion that the successful evaluation of a course prepares for the eventuality of a more successful subsequent course. What the course chairman is ultimately responsible for is to "determine whether the design and delivery of a program were effective and whether the proposed outcomes were met" [2].

## 2.9    Managing the course and avoiding common pitfalls (12–6 months in advance)

The role of the course chairman in managing the planning process is one of constant oversight, setting priorities, and coordinating the completion of tasks taken on by the team. The task of developing a course from initial concept through to fruition is difficult. Initial themes, preliminary assessment of learner needs, and the introduction of new medical advances that drove the initial planning when the course was established will not come to fruition without constant effort. New ideas, which can improve upon an old course, will not come to pass unless there is a successful plan put in place to make change happen. Special initiatives for individual courses must be carefully worked upon in a collaborative fashion with the entire planning team to ensure thoughts and ideas can and do flourish. In North America, new electronic communication for course production has helped a great deal to establish collaboration, connectivity, and cooperation among faculty. The "eRoom" has revolutionized the ability to put on a course with a paperless initial planning process by allowing for the discussion of thoughts, ideas, and concepts among a large audience of faculty before the course takes place. The target for courses is to have an agreed-on preplan established at least one year in advance.

The course chairman must always be prepared for and try to prevent course pitfalls. It is not unusual for one to two invited speakers in a large course (40 faculty persons) to be unavailable because of some personal or professional crisis. This reality must be taken into consideration, and a plan put in place to deal with it if it occurs. Other eventualities that need to be anticipated and planned for include:

- Resource insufficiency.
- Falling behind on time-lines.
- Weather-related emergencies.
- Political upheavals **(Table 2-2)**.

The chairman needs to challenge the rest of the team to anticipate possible problems, as well as create contingency plans to deal with them.

Table 2-2a    **Algorithm (for Switzerland) for carrying out AO courses in territories of war or high risk**

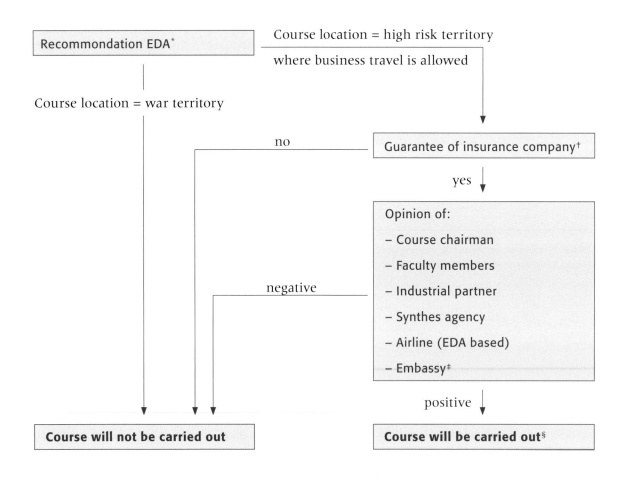

* EDA is the Swiss Federal Department for Foreign Affairs, www.eda.admin.ch
† For certain areas a guarantee of the respective insurance company must be given prior to departure.
‡ Recommended to register in embassy in course territory.
§ For any business travel the respective AO collaborator has to sign an agreement of consent.
The respective business travels will internally be approved by the associated institutional head.

Table 2-2b    **Checklist for carrying out an AO course in**

City: _____    Country: _____    Date: _____

| Recommondation EDA* | Course location = war territory | ▨ |
|---|---|---|
| | Business travel is allowed | ☐ |
| Date: | No limitation in travelling mentioned | ☐ |

| Guarantee of insurance company† | Declined | ▨ |
|---|---|---|
| | Is given but with restrictions | ☐ |
| Date: | Is given | ☐ |

Opinion of:                                                                 Carry out    Cancel

| | | | | Carry out | Cancel |
|---|---|---|---|---|---|
| Course chairman | Name: | | Date: | ☐ | ☐ |
| Faculty members | Name: | | Date: | ☐ | ☐ |
| | Name: | | Date: | ☐ | ☐ |
| Industrial partner | Name: | | Date: | ☐ | ☐ |
| Synthes agency | Name: | | Date: | ☐ | ☐ |
| Airline (EDA based) | Name: | | Date: | ☐ | ☐ |
| Embassy‡ | Name: | | Date: | ☐ | ☐ |

| If any ☐ field is filled in, the course will not be carried out. | The final decision has to be taken by AOI on the basis of the above recommendations. |
|---|---|
| | Decision: ☐ yes    ☐ no |
| | Date: _____ Signature: _____ |

* EDA is the Swiss Federal Department for Foreign Affairs, www.eda.admin.ch

† For certain areas a guarantee of the respective insurance company must be given prior to departure.

‡ Recommended to register in embassy in course territory.

### 2.10 Completing planning and logistical details (6–3 months in advance)

As the course approaches, the tasks of the chairman shift to attending to more detailed planning issues. Although the basic essentials and structure of the course have been established, specific issues usually develop around timing of the course, course flow, handouts, possible new content, electronic communications with participants and faculty, team building, and/or leadership issues. Each of these issues must be dealt with when it arises and in a way that does not interfere with other aspects of the course.

### 2.11 Collaborating with other chairmen (6–3 months in advance)

Course chairmen should work collaboratively to share with each other progress on tasks in order to provide the best possible course. It is easy to have a course go astray because the course chairmen themselves do not necessarily work cooperatively in a fashion that is synergistic. Coordination of courses is vital, if, for example, there are only facilities to run practicals at one given time. Providing formal or informal status reports to each other can often uncover potential problems not seen by one course chairman alone. Sharing the specifics of a problem that suddenly occurred helps a course chairman obtain valuable input about possible solutions that are usually better than what might be developed by one chair acting unilaterally. Also, hearing about new developments in another course might suggest enhancements that should be considered for the course being planned.

### 3 Planning the precourse faculty meeting

The precourse is a vital part of all AO courses. This activity involves all the faculty and staff and is chaired by the course chairman and usually occurs shortly before the start of the actual course. It is generally agreed that the degree of success of the actual course is directly related to the effectiveness of the precourse. The primary purpose of this session is to provide faculty with all the information that would be helpful in better understanding the nature of their audience such as skill level, geographic differences, age, and years since residency. In addition, the course chairman can also describe the overall course and how each faculty presentation, small group activity, and panel discussion fits into the larger picture. Providing this information for faculty helps to assure that the outcome-based learning objectives are met [12]. An effective plan for the precourse by the course chairman will set the stage for the course to flow more effectively.

■ ▫ **The better the precourse, the more successful the actual course will be.**

Every seasoned course chairman has experienced a course that began without a precourse or with a poor precourse. As a result, the designed learning experience was not implemented in a manner consistent with what was necessary to meet the objectives and the course began to unravel on the first day. The participants in such a course usually sense disarray quickly, which further adds to the growing problem.

Faculty should come to the venue with a relatively firm idea regarding their role within the course. The precourse carefully outlines those roles and ensures that prior to the course there are no questions about the roles of individual faculty in each of the different educational formats and methods designed for the participants. Faculty members need to be made aware of course objectives, themes, special learning formats that are being introduced, or communication technologies that are designed to enhance learning. A cohesive group of faculty is more likely to present information in a more effective fashion and not contradict one another or deliver information in very different fashions.

■ ▦    **A precourse can also establish a sense of teamwork and morale for the faculty. Faculty who are focused, and who teach with a deliberate and efficacious style, in a repetitive and reinforcing fashion should enhance participants' learning experience.**

The precourse is extremely important to the delivery of an effective educational experience. It should be organized by the chairman to outline each component of the course in a systematic fashion, including the lecture, the laboratory, and the small group discussion components. Other administrative requirements such as course location, break and meal times, start and ending times need to be covered in the precourse. The constant mantra used by the AO is "failing to plan is planning to fail". This is used repetitively within all AO courses and it speaks volumes about the important role of the course chairman.

## 4    During the course

The course chairmen need to arrive at the course early to survey the actual site for the course and to start the troubleshooting process. The precourse talk itself needs to be prepared in advance to emphasize the quality of the event, the leadership behind it, and the expectations for all involved. The challenge of the chairman is to:

- Attempt to encourage the best of a positive faculty spirit **(Fig 2-4)**.
- Infuse energy into the event.
- Constantly articulate the course themes and objectives.
- Provide learning pearls to the participants.
- Do everything humanly possible to prevent any pitfalls or problems.

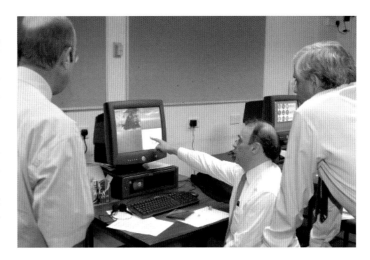

Fig 2-4    Fully equipped faculty room for them to prepare, discuss, and also relax.

This establishes a solid rapport with faculty, industrial partner staff, and the other chairmen. All aspects of the course need to have back-up plans. A continuous two-way feedback system needs to be worked out with the administrative staff to ensure that the course runs smoothly. Course chairmen need to be able to react to the local physical, academic, and personal environment to better meet the needs of those that are working to make this a memorable event.

Another important quality of a successful course chairman is effective leadership. Certain individuals demonstrate leadership with their personal flair, dedication, and spirit. It is not necessarily the most senior faculty, or the person with the most publications who makes the best course chairman. Characteristics of a successful course chairman fall into categories of organizational skills, time management efficiency, and ability to cooperate, collaborate, and synthesize with all involved participants on the planning team. Problems of communication, effective education, and resource utilization should be anticipated. Said simply, the course chairman needs to be:

- A leader.
- A communicator.
- A collaborator.
- An organizer.
- A positive thinker.

A course chairman must think of last-minute ways to best use all physical, human, and intellectual resources to maximize the educational experience of those at the course. Often, last minute changes can be made during the course as a reaction to focus groups or feedback which occurs on site. Course chairmen also need to identify something unique about everyone involved in implementing the course, to spread praise, and to be positive. Lastly, the course chairman should thank those who have helped in planning and implementing the course, especially the support staff (**Fig 2-5**) who have worked so diligently for months and throughout the actual course.

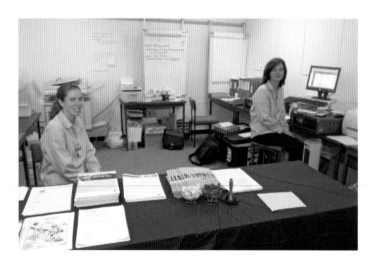

Fig 2-5    Supporting staff need to create a fully equipped office at the course site.

## 5    After the course

After the course has concluded, several additional re-sponsibilities need to be carried out by the course chair-man, within the first week:

- Evaluate the course.
- Complete unfinished administrative details.
- Provide formal thank-you notes.
- Complete report on suggested enhancements.
- Communicate with the next course chairman.

Feedback from a course will quickly be forgotten if it is not captured quickly during and immediately after a course. Thoughts, impressions, and individual feelings are very important to the next course chairman and this must be recorded to establish a report of the positive and negative aspects of the course and suggested enhance-ments. It is suggested that during the course, the course chairman write down thoughts and impressions on a daily basis, so that these can be summarized to pass on to future course chairmen.

The course chairmen and administrative staff need to quickly summarize the evaluations for a course. These data are critical to understanding what worked and what did not and which objectives were and were not met. In addition to reading through summarized evaluation data, the planning team also needs to start the analysis of these data. The course chairman needs to be a part of this process to assist in the transmission of this impor-tant information to the next chairman. The end result of this process is the creation of a final course report for the AO staff and the next course chairman.

One of the enhancements to this process that AO is be-ginning to implement is a follow-up (3–6 months after the course) evaluation of a sampling of participants. The purpose of this will be to better understand the degree to which the course objectives were met and the desired behavioral outcomes were reached by the participants. The outcomes of this effort are used for decision making and accountability by using the results for:

- Improving the design and implementation of the course.
- Understanding how the course participants are using the information provided and skills taught back in their practice setting.
- Studying the impact of political, geographic, and other organizational variables on course success.
- Making suggestions for changes in the next course.
- Obtaining additional learning needs for additional courses.

The essence of this effort is to determine the ultimate worth of the educational venture [2].

The process of critically analyzing the course not only yields data about how to improve the next one, it also uncovers certain individuals who went above and be-yond expectations to assure a quality learning experi-ence. These individuals need to be recognized and thanked by the chairman. Also, the regional develop-ment of potential new faculty and possible new chair-men is of great significance. Without careful local, national, and international collaboration and coopera-tion, the future course chairmen will be reinventing the wheel, rather than building on what has succeeded in the past.

## 6 Conclusion

A successful course can be measured by many factors.

The **first** factor is the warmth and good feelings that occur as the course unfolds on a day-to-day basis. Immediate feedback from participants and faculty will filter to the course chairman and often provides the message that all of the work that has gone into the planning of a course has been worthwhile. Course chairmen are volunteers and they need to hear positive feedback to continue to provide their stewardship.

**Secondly**, evaluations from participants and faculty need to be seen by the course chairmen so that they can learn from the process. Administrative staff is invaluable in this particular instance. The continuous and repetitive process of putting on courses allows for each course to build upon past good events.

**Thirdly**, excitement generated in participants by the course is evident when they return home and disseminate knowledge about AO, its techniques, and new surgical procedures. Also, if they had a successful educational experience, they will likely return for another AO course or join the AO network.

**Lastly**, course participants will have been provided with data on new surgical procedures and tools to assess the continuous quality improvement of their practice. The importance of AO educators and mentors at local institutions cannot be understated. The knowledge, skill, and attitude learned at an AO course and the enthusiasm generated by that course provide the gold standard for patient care.

■ ▪ **The essence of being a successful AO course chairman is that delivery of a gold-standard AO course lives on in improved patient care.**

## 7    Anecdote

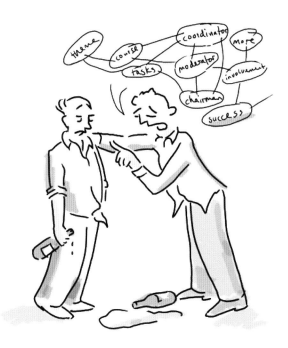

*Positive things can happen when course coordinators work well together. An example of this was the first course that I was acting as a course chairman. My co-course organizer was also new at this task, but we sat down over one or two good stiff drinks and spent about 6 hours planning our course fully 1 ½ years before its eventual occurrence. This 6-hour meeting laid a strong foundation with structure, themes, and careful coordination of tasks. We decided on a new direction for our course with more involvement of moderators, and this was emphasized through the whole course. We also agreed upon a theme—example: evidence-based medicine, and we strongly encouraged faculty to be involved in this particular course direction. This also was very successful when the course eventually came to fruition. The initial 6 hours that we spent also established a good rapport between the two of us so that each of us knew exactly which tasks the other one was involved with doing. A strong working relationship developed, and we had a very successful and well-coordinated course because of this initial meeting which was over a bar stool in a foreign country. Positive vibrations can come from good communication and this particular 6-hour discussion was extremely fruitful.*

*Rick Buckley*

## 8 Bibliography

1. **Grosswald SJ** (1984) Designing effective educational activities for groups. *Green JS, Grosswald SJ, Suter E, et al (eds). Continuing Education for the Health Professions: Developing, Managing and Evaluating Programs for Maximum Impact on Patient Care.* San Francisco: Jossey-Bass Publishers, 175.
2. **Caffarella RS** (2002) *Planning Programs for Adult Learners.* San Francisco: Jossey-Bass, John Wiley & Sons.
3. **Pennington F, Green JS** (1976) Comparative analysis of program development processes in six professions. *Adult Education;* 27(1): 13–23.
4. **Conner DR** (1998) *Leading at the Edge of Chaos: How to Create the Nimble Organization.* New York: John Wiley & Sons Inc.
5. **Moon J** (2004) Using reflective learning to improve the impact of short courses and workshops. *J Contin Edu Health Prof;* 24(1):5–7.
6. **Lundy J** (1994) *TEAMS: How to Develop Peak Performance Teams for World-Class Results.* Chicago: Dartnell.
7. **Lockyer J** (2003) Performance of health professionals to determine priorities and shape interventions. *Davis DA, Barnes BE, Fox RD (eds). The Continuing Professional Development of Physicians: From Research to Practice.* Chicago: AMA Press.
8. **Knox AB** (1965) *Clientele analysis. Review of Educational Research;* 35(3):231–239.
9. **Campbell C** (2003) Identifying the needs of the individual learner. *Davis DA, Barnes BE, Fox RD (eds). The Continuing Professional Development of Physicians: From Research to Practice.* Chicago: AMA Press.
10. **Prochaska JO, DiClemente CC** (1983) Stages and process of self-change of smoking: toward an integration model of change. *Journal of Consulting and Clinical Psychology;* 51(3):390–395.
11. **Casebeer L, Centor RM, Kristofco RE** (2003) Learning in large and small groups. *Davis DA, Barnes BE, Fox RD (eds). The Continuing Professional Development of Physicians: From Research to Practice.* Chicago: AMA Press.
12. **Suter E, Green JS, Grosswald SJ, et al** (1984) Introduction: defining quality for continuing education. *Green JS, Grosswald SJ, Suter E, et al (eds). Continuing Education for the Health Professions: Developing, Managing and Evaluating Programs for Maximum Impact on Patient Care.* San Francisco: Jossey-Bass Publishers, 25.

Authors   Roger KJ Simmermacher, John R Kues

# 3   How to run a discussion group

## 1   Introduction

Talking about cases is an important part of AO courses. Course faculty and course participants have always felt free to bring x-rays of their own patients to share and discuss together. Initially, these talks were conversation-based on the assumption that people accept statements on trust and mutual respect. However, to be of educational value, discussions must rely on the provision of arguments supported by evidence and proven criteria. Case discussions are useful for supporting one's preformed opinions and can elicit new thoughts on a difficult clinical case. Discussions also allow course participants to test their new knowledge gained at lectures and the opportunity for additional clarification on learning points from the faculty.

■ ▦   **Discussion groups are cornerstones in AO teaching. Evidence-based case discussions are key to apply the learning outcome in daily practice.**

Several years ago, planned "fire-side" discussions were introduced into the official program of some courses in order to discuss the principles of fracture management in small groups using cases delivered by an appointed discussion leader. These sessions did not attain their intended goals due to a lack of structure and inadequate planning by the faculty. It was decided, however, that this method of learning was very valuable and needed to be permanently integrated into AO courses.

This chapter provides the reader with some guidelines to help optimize the learning potential of discussion groups and to improve the satisfaction of both course participants and faculty. We recognize that each learn-

ing situation is unique, and the suggestions in this chapter will need to be adapted to fit different venues, group sizes, and socio-demographic compositions.

■ ▦   **By the end of this chapter the reader should be able to:**

▦   **Organize a small discussion group meeting.**
▦   **Realize that the discussion leader is more moderator than lecturer.**
▦   **Realize that preparation is of importance.**
▦   **Realize that there are some pitfalls.**

## 1.1   Goal of a discussion within the course

In the context of courses, discussions are faculty-led exchanges among a group of participants. The exchanges are focused on clinical cases and are meant to reinforce information that is covered in the course lectures and practical exercises (practicals). From the point of view of an outside observer or course participant, discussion sessions may appear to be a free exchange of opinion and information. However, although discussion groups may appear to be loose and informal, there is a great deal of organization and preparation necessary to ensure that they achieve their objectives. To be successful, discussions should promote the open exchange of thoughts and ideas about the case being presented [1].

Depending on the type of course (principles, advances, or masters) the goal of a small discussion group varies. Most of the course participants in an AO Principles Course are junior or senior surgical trainees. They have limited experience, and this course is providing them with some basic theoretical background. Trainees at this type of course tend to be young, and many of them may have limited knowledge of the language in which the course is being taught. As a result, active participation in a small group discussion may be difficult and they may be hesitant to share their thoughts and questions. There are two important goals for discussion groups in the AO Principles Courses. The first goal is to develop a stronger sense of understanding with regard to the diagnosis and treatment techniques covered by the course. Course participants should feel confident in their knowledge and ability to discuss cases with colleagues and faculty. The second goal is to be able to apply theories presented during lectures and practicals in discussions about real clinical cases. A successful discussion group at a AO Principles Course results in participants that can organize their thoughts and can step through decision-making exercises with a group of comparable colleagues while trying to solve clinical problems.

■ ▥   **The discussion leader of an AO Principles Course in these groups should be aware of the fact that, at this level, the participants still expect some expert information from them. It is important that leaders skillfully guide the discussion without lecturing to the participants.**

Many of the same principles apply for small discussion groups held during AO Advances Courses. They are also intended to create an atmosphere in which course participants can initiate case discussions based on their own experience and new information from the course lectures. Participants normally are at least senior surgical trainees, but mostly (young) consultants and experienced at presenting their own ideas.

Discussion groups held during experts' meetings essentially should be what the ancient Greeks called a "symposium". All participants are at the same level and thesis and antithesis should finally end in synthesis based upon respect and appreciation of others' ideas and rationales developed according to a specific case. AO discussion groups—unlike Greek symposia—usually do not involve alcohol. However, as previously stated, the attitude demonstrated by the discussion leaders should always be one of creating an atmosphere of mutual respect for the thoughts presented. Irrespective of the level of the participants, the group leaders' style is crucial for the success of the meeting [2–4]. This means that sometimes the choice between a more controlled discussion, intended to solve a problem, and a more open discussion, which is more reflective and leads to new ideas, has to be made as the leader watches the group dynamics unfold during the session [3].

■ ▥   **A discussion group creates an atmosphere wherein:**

   ▥ **There is mutual respect for thoughts presented.**
   ▥ **Participants develop a sense of self-efficacy with regard to their own possibilities to interpret cases.**
   ▥ **Participants learn to apply theoretical knowledge presented in the lectures on cases.**

## 2    A discussion in a small group

The leader of the discussion group should preferably be an active consultant with some years of experience, although this might depend on the type of course. The more experienced the group of course participants is, the more the role of the discussion leader changes from director to moderator. With younger participants the discussion leader needs to direct a discussion among the course participants and to involve them in it. In this environment, the role of the discussion leader is primarily to help them organize their own thoughts and link them to thoughts expressed by others. This process is more critical and time-consuming in groups of inexperienced course participants than in more advanced groups. The difference in experience between the discussion leader and course participants allows the leader to have more control and makes it somewhat easier to be more directive in facilitating discussions. In more experienced groups, however, the discussion is likely to be more spontaneous. The challenge for the leader in these groups is to keep the discussion focused on the issues of the specific case at hand. Redirecting unrelated discussions—while allowing relevant issues to emerge—requires skillful facilitation so as not to dominate the group. Finally, the discussion leader(s) should be thoroughly familiar with the issues of the case so that they can adapt to any direction the course participants take the discussion.

The discussion group leader generally should be aware of the basic principles of adult learning as pointed out in other chapters of this book (eg, 2 How to be a course chairman and 6 How to give a lecture) and at least adhere to the principle of set, dialogue, and closure. Ability to listen to the course participants and to reformulate their remarks into either open- or closed-ended questions will improve the likelihood of involving more people in an active discussion [1–5].

■ ▦    **It is also very important for the discussion leaders to avoid presenting their own successes in difficult cases and to restrain from dogmatic statements based solely on their own experience.**

As the accepted expert, these kinds of assertions are likely to eliminate other opinions or solutions and can stifle discussion [4].

Generally, 45–60 minutes appear to be the maximum length of most discussion groups. Although the level of concentration of all participants is influenced by the time of the day, it is hard to imagine that more than three cases can be thoroughly discussed in a single session. This means that the targeted time for completing a discussion of a case should be approximately 15 minutes.

### 2.1    Before the course

It is always much easier to prepare for a discussion group if the cases are chosen beforehand. The cases for discussion should closely parallel the information presented in the lectures. Typically, four to six cases should be selected for discussion sessions that are scheduled for 45–60 minutes. That number allows for one or two extra cases in the event that a case does not work well or if the group moves rapidly through each case. In order to have all course participants discussing the same cases, not necessarily in the same order, the organizing committee of a course should select appropriate cases with the information necessary and send them to the discussion leaders in advance of the course. The cases chosen should be consistent with the new theoretical knowledge and should not show significant deviations or curious solutions. In expert groups it may be possible to allow the introduction of participants' own cases. Participant-selected cases may widen the range of discussion but it also requires the discussion leader to be especially attentive to the overall objectives of the discussion session. Using preselected cases has the advantage of allowing the discussion leader to stratify the discussion according to the themes of the day (such material can be obtained on CD-ROM through AO International). Each case should contain a general description of the patient and the circumstances of the injury. X-rays should be presented whenever possible. In most cases, multiple x-rays are desirable. When cases are constructed it may be useful to provide the discussion group leaders with complete information and an abbreviated presentation of the case may be prepared for presentation in the discussion group.

Ideally, each small discussion group should have two facilitators. One faculty member should take responsibility for facilitating the discussion while the other plays a supportive role. The faculty member in the supportive role can operate the audiovisual (AV) equipment, pass out any handout materials, operate x-ray view boxes or models, and provide an additional expert opinion. This frees the other faculty member to describe the case, prompt the group with questions, and keep the discussion focused. Faculty members should agree on their roles prior to the beginning of the discussion session. Faculty members may switch roles between cases to allow each the opportunity to play both roles. Faculty members may negotiate different roles from those depicted above but the roles should be clear and have minimal overlap. The role of each faculty member should also be described to the course participants so there is no confusion. Generally both faculty members should be facilitating and not dominating.

■ ▥ **Roles of the two faculty members for small discussion groups:**
**Role 1—facilitator, ie, case presenter, discussion moderator.**
**Role 2—supporter, eg, operating AV, distribute handouts, etc.**

The venue of a small discussion group might be most variable and largely depends on the location of the course. The ideal number of participants is between six and eight and the room should accommodate the maximum number of participants comfortably. Distractions like the noise of a neighboring discussion group or trespassing staff members should be kept to a minimum. The configuration of the seating should allow easy eye contact among all the participants. A circular arrangement is optimal, however, since x-rays or slides will typically be presented a horseshoe configuration of the chairs might be more practical [3, 4] **(Fig 3-1)**. In this case the faculty facilitator should be located at the open end of the horseshoe with their back facing the screen. When discussing a slide or x-ray the discussion leader should stand to the side so that all course participants can see the screen.

It's always advisable to test the AV tools prior to the beginning of the discussion session. All of the x-rays and other slides should be readily available to make it easy to move from one presentation to the next. If a computerized slide show is used for presenting case materials, all case materials should be preloaded onto the computer where they are easily identified and can be quickly

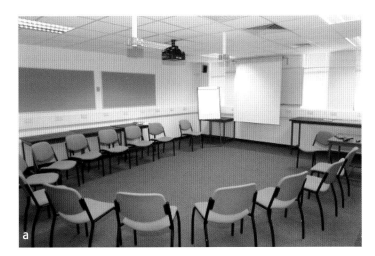 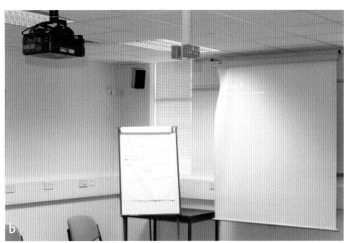

Fig 3-1a–b    A classical horseshoe-like configuration and equipment for a discussion group of about 10–12 participants.

accessed. If a flipchart is available, this might be quite helpful to explain more abstract issues with the help of a drawing. If a flipchart will be used heavily, it is useful to have a role of tape available so that pages can be torn from the chart pad and taped on a nearby wall, or other structure, so that multiple pages can be viewed simultaneously. Room lighting can become a difficult issue when using x-rays and slides. In order to properly view many visual aids the lights need to be lowered. However, discussions are difficult to conduct when participants cannot easily see each other. A room should be selected in which it is possible to adjust the lighting. The ideal lighting situation is one in which lights near the screen or x-ray box can be turned down or off while leaving the rest of the room reasonably well lit. If such an arrangement is not available, the most viable alternative is a room with lights that can be dimmed. The most difficult room situation is one in which the lights can only be turned completely off or on. In this type of room it may be necessary to turn off the lights to view specific slides and then turn them back on to continue discussion. Having slides that are relatively easy to read in fully lighted rooms is the best way to reduce problems due to lighting. High-contrast slides (very dark background and white print or white background and very dark print) work best in this situation. Of equal concern, but more difficult to control, is the temperature of the room. Arriving to a room early may give you enough time to have the temperature adjusted in time for the discussion session. Finally, your mobile telephone and those of the course participants should be switched off.

A laptop computer with a projector and a screen is ideal but might not be possible. X-ray view boxes to present x-rays are an alternative but may create problems due to limited visibility. Lengthy, detailed PowerPoint presentations should be avoided since they can rapidly become a lecture. Instead, simple but clear illustration of the problem to be discussed should be used. Essential information should be given at an early stage either orally or with some key words on the slide to easily start a discussion. If it is practical, physical models may be used. They have the advantage of being "low tech" and can allow the kind of 3-D views that are not typically available on x-rays. They also eliminate all of the problems that were previously described with room lighting.

## 2.2 At the precourse

It is vital that the information to be presented in the discussion groups is made available to the discussion group leaders before the course. Ideally, this can be sent to them as a CD-ROM before the precourse. The material on the CD-ROM would be the images to be shown to the course participants and an information sheet showing the learning aims and objectives of each presentation.

■ ▥ **Cases to be presented together with individual learning aims and objectives are submitted to the discussion group leaders well in advance so that they can be discussed at the precourse.**

The material needs to be discussed at the precourse to make sure that all the discussion group leaders agree that the material to be presented is suitable. The precourse is also the opportunity for the discussion group leaders to openly debate any areas of disagreement that they may have about the treatment options that are being shown to the course participants. It is much better if a single-agreed policy can be settled at this time. Overt or covert disagreements that become public during the course undermine the credibility of the faculty members and confuse the course participants.

## 2.3 During the course

The meeting should begin with the introduction of the two discussion leaders. A brief biographical presentation that includes current titles and position along with a brief background is sufficient for this purpose. If the group is small (six to eight course participants) you may ask participants to introduce themselves and where they are from. One of the discussion leaders should explain the overall purpose of the discussion group. This should include the role of the group leaders and any ground rules for discussions [2, 4].

■ ▥ **Ground rules:**

▥ **Establish roles of faculty members.**
▥ **Establish roles for course participants: participation is essential, there are no bad questions, discourage early closure on discussion items.**
▥ **Prevent faculty from answering the questions before course participants do.**
▥ **Faculty person to provide summary and synthesis at the end of each case.**

For example, you might tell the participants that cases will be briefly described and then an open discussion, with questions and comments, will proceed for approximately 15 minutes; then the discussion leader will bring the case discussion to a close with a summary of the learning points. Each case should be presented with a brief introduction that includes a description of the patient and the circumstances of the injury. This information can be summarized in one or two slides or in a brief handout. X-rays, photographs, and other audiovisuals should be briefly presented and described. It can be helpful, especially in groups with younger, less experienced participants, to present two or three succinct questions in order to help focus the discussion. Each case should be a complete and independent learning experience. This format prevents unforeseen interruptions or cases that extend well beyond their allotted time from compromising the setting of the whole meeting. The set-dialogue-closure model should be consistently used for all cases in order to maintain some consistency in the overall session.

It is important to get the course participants actively engaged as early as possible in the discussion session. If the group is small, the leader can facilitate this by learning the names of the participants and asking their opinion or comment on an early discussion question [3, 5]. With larger groups you can engage the course participants early by asking them to respond to a question by raising their hands or verbally agreeing or disagreeing.

■ ▦    **Questions like "How many of you have seen a case like this?" or "How many of you would use technique A? and How many would use technique B?", etc can be used to engage the participants.**

Discussion can be greatly enhanced if you can encourage participants to direct questions to the group instead of to the discussion leader [3].

■ ▦    **The faculty member can model this behavior by turning questions back to the group with comments like, "What do the rest of you think about this?" or "How have the rest of you dealt with this issue in your practice?"**

Obviously, this technique works better in discussion groups with more experienced participants. Faculty members should be careful not to allow discussions among course participants to become too unrelated to the case or the learning goals.

In small groups, eye contact with the participants can be very important to facilitating discussion by everyone. Even somewhat shy participants will feel motivated to say something if the discussion leader continues to look directly at them. Many participants who are shy or have difficulty speaking the language of the meeting may show that they are learning by nonverbal cues. For example, they may nod their head to signal that they agree with a point or that they understand something that was said. It may be possible to increase their participation by asking them a direct question or by inviting everyone to respond to a particular question. For example, after a statement is made the discussion leader may ask everyone to indicate their agreement or disagreement with what was said. If the group is small, the discussion leader may ask everyone to comment on their vote. However, it is not critical that the faculty member get everyone to actively participate in the discussion. Quite early it will be apparent whether the discussion needs to be fueled by the faculty member or whether the participants themselves will assure discussion. Typically, faculty members will notice that there are "talkers" (extroverts) and "listeners" (introverts) in the group. Extroverts tend to think and learn as they are speaking. Introverts, on the other hand, learn best by taking time to reflect on what was said [1]. Short discussions of 10–15 minutes may be sufficient time to allow introverts to reflect on early points that were made and to participate toward the end of the case. If several cases focus on one general theme you are more likely to have active participation by the introverts in the group.

■ ▦ **Extroverts tend to think and learn while they are speaking—introverts learn by reflecting on what was said.**

The faculty member should be careful not to allow the discussion to be dominated by one or two course participants. There are several ways in which this might happen. A particularly eager learner may ask repeated questions that require detailed answers. If the faculty member can acknowledge that these are good questions and ask the other participants to offer answers, the dominant participant can be turned into an asset for group discussion. A second scenario is one in which the course participants see themselves as experts and attempt to provide definitive answers to all questions. The discussion leader can acknowledge that the answer is a good one but that there are other answers or solutions that are also possible. The discussion leader can then ask other members of the group to suggest alternatives. If a course participant attempts to dominate the group discussion by repeatedly engaging the discussion leader in a one-on-one conversation, the faculty member might suggest that this issue requires more time than has been allotted for the case under discussion and that the leader would be happy to continue the discussion with that group member at a later time in order to stay on time [4].

If the seating arrangement in the discussion group is an open horseshoe with the discussion group leader at one end of it, the person who has the most eye contact with the discussion group leader is the participant in the center of the horseshoe. This is the so-called "position of influence", the seat next to the group discussion group leader has no eye contact with the discussion group leader and the participant in that seat is the one least likely to participate in the discussion. Placing a course participant who is attempting to dominate the group into the seat next to the discussion group leader is a strategy worth considering. Placing a course participant who is reluctant to get involved in the seat of influence may also facilitate more discussion.

■ ▦ **The leader should take the last minute or two of each case discussion to summarize the key learning points that were made. These should be closely linked to the initial learning objectives for the case and should be consistent with the general learning points that have been made in lectures and practicals.**

### 2.3.1 Dangers and problems

There are many potential problem issues that may occur during small group discussion sessions. Some of these have been discussed in other chapters and most of them can be overcome if the discussion leaders are prepared and recognize the problems early. A lack of preparation creates the largest risk for problems in any educational situation. Discussion group sessions are particularly susceptible to problems because they are open and lack the structure that exists in lectures and other educational formats [3].

■ ▥    **Knowing the learning objectives and having a thorough familiarity with the cases are probably the two most critical areas of preparation.**

If a discussion leader can master these two areas of preparation they should have no difficulty providing a good educational experience for the course participants.

Facilitation skills are probably the next most important factor for success and avoiding problems. While many of the points made in this chapter can be very helpful in addressing problems that arise, experience over time will improve overall facilitation skills. The main purpose of discussion groups is to allow participants to test their knowledge and to clarify points that have been made in the lectures and practicals. The use of real cases as focal points for discussion is a very powerful learning tool if the participants are actively engaged. These groups are not designed as a forum for leaders to demonstrate their expertise or to attempt to change the attitudes of the participants. The leader's role is to promote discussion in a safe, respectful, and enthusiastic environment [5]. As ambassadors for AO, the discussion leader should be professional and respectful of all participants. Demeaning comments, inappropriate jokes, and statements that could be interpreted as sexual or racial harassment should never be used or tolerated in the group.

Techniques that work in one group may not work in another group. Group size, the level of expertise, and the personalities of the participants can determine which facilitation techniques work best. In small groups (less than eight people) it is usually easier to get all participants to become actively engaged in discussion [3, 4].

Since non-participation is very conspicuous in groups of this size, there is a great deal of pressure on each individual to comment or ask a question. In larger groups, discussion leaders may notice that up to 25% of the group may not actively participate. It is more difficult to identify each individual and to use techniques like eye contact to encourage them to participate. In addition, the relatively short amount of time devoted to each case makes it more difficult to maintain discussions long enough to allow everyone to ask a question or make a comment.

Larger groups are more susceptible to multiple simultaneous discussions. "Buzz" groups are smaller, two-to-four-person groups, that begin a conversation among themselves while the remaining members of the group continue their general discussion [1, 2, 4]. Sometimes it is possible to bring the buzz-group discussion into the larger group while waiting 5–10 seconds before continuing the larger group discussion. If that is unsuccessful you might acknowledge the buzz-group discussion and ask them to continue their conversation at a later time in order for the large group discussion to stay on time.

In case of language problems, especially if native and nonnative speakers are in one group, it is difficult to keep the pace of discussion. There are certainly people who will not get any message due to a near complete lack of the language spoken but intense observation will identify those who might be involved in the discussion if the pace is slowed. Furthermore, repetition of the key words of a message will help to make opinions more understandable. This technique should be used as early as possible so as not to lose the course participants who are struggling to understand the discussion. Sometimes it is helpful to ask at the beginning who is a native speaker and who is not. Other members of the group may speak slower or use simpler words and phrases to help the nonnative speakers. Leaders should watch the nonnative speakers more carefully in order to detect signs that they may not be following the discussion.

■ ▦ **Repetition of the key words of a message help to make opinions understandable.**

Another strategy worth trying is to split the group into smaller groups according to their native language. Each group can be allocated a case to discuss and after 10 minutes or so, the participant with the best linguistic skills can be asked to present their groups conclusions. The discussion group leader will usually find that there is at least one member of each language group who has reasonable linguistic skills.

## 2.4 After the course

Formal evaluation of discussion groups with forms is usually unhelpful. Therefore, personal contact with the participants directly after the meeting or during the tea/coffee breaks will help to identify how the discussion group could have been better. One should not expect too much feedback from this technique but it will tell whether certain goals were met. One very useful mechanism of evaluation is a discussion between the two discussion group leaders. Identifying which tech-

niques were successful and which were not can help the leaders make adjustments for the future. Additionally, senior discussion leaders should take time with junior leaders to critique their performance and offer suggestions. During analysis one should clarify whether the learning objectives were well explained and met, whether the set-dialogue-closure scheme was followed and whether measures have to be taken to address problems that occurred (eg, repositioning several discussants or even taking somebody aside if his behavior was disruptive for the rest of the group). Finally, sometimes, fellow faculty members who observed the meeting are a valuable source of additional information [2].

■ ▦ **A small AO discussion group should:**

▦ **Be well prepared concerning case selection, timing, and venue.**
▦ **Follow the set-dialogue-closure layout format.**
▦ **Seek to actively engage the participants.**
▦ **Be moderated, not presented.**
▦ **Reinforce the basic educational messages of the overall course.**

## 3    A discussion in a large group

Discussion groups of 40 or more participants are almost an oxymoron since the large numbers make it virtually impossible to conduct a discussion among all the attendees. However, it is possible to apply many of the principles described earlier in this chapter to facilitate good interaction among participants and the group leaders. Many of the rules in the chapter on presenting a lecture (see 6 How to give a lecture; 3 During the course) are useful, especially the ones concerning eye contact and body language. If the large discussion group is primarily intended as an informal way to summarize the main learning objectives of the entire course it is helpful to have a team of three faculty members leading the discussion. It will then be a presentation of that group of faculty that actively tries to get at least part of the course participants to make comments and ask questions. Cases representing the main issues of the course should be carefully selected prior to the discussion. Each of the two or more faculty members/discussion group leaders should present one case. A clear delineation of roles for each of the faculty members should be planned just as it would be done for a small group discussion.

■ ▥    **In the large group, unlike the small group, it requires at least three faculty members to maintain good eye contact and to observe body language across the entire group of course participants.**

The educational experience of the discussion leaders is much less critical for large group discussions than it is for a small group discussion. The educational experience level of almost any faculty member at an AO course should be sufficient to direct a large group discussion.

Faculty members must however be sufficiently clinically experienced to answer any questions. Prior experience as a lecturer is an advantage when facilitating a large group discussion since they will have some familiarity with the skills necessary to keep the attention of a large audience. In general, only faculty who have experience in giving lectures and facilitating large group discussions are likely to volunteer for this kind of assignment **(Fig 3-2)**. It is not advisable to appoint inexperienced or unwilling faculty to this duty. New faculty members who want to gain experience can be given responsibilities as support faculty member and may serve as co-leader to a large group discussion session with a more experienced faculty member.

It is more difficult to hold the attention of a large group for long periods of time. For that reason it is advisable that large group discussion sessions be scheduled for shorter amounts of time than small group discussions. Typically, 45 minutes is the maximum time for which a large group discussion should be scheduled. As with small group discussions, each case should be presented, discussed, and summarized in 12–15 minutes. This can present a challenge to the discussion leader(s) since the larger number of course participants often means that there are more questions and opinions.

Faculty members have a choice as to the opinions they express with regard to the treatment of the cases that are presented. Faculty members can agree in advance to take a particular line regardless of how they feel about the management of a given case. Such a policy leads to a lively debate but from the participants point of view it is probably best to allow faculty members to express their true clinical opinion.

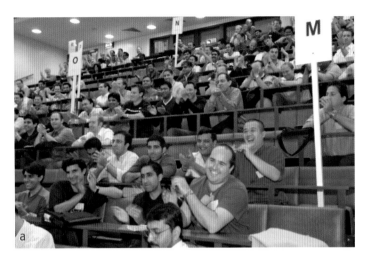
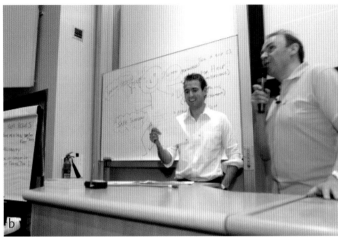

Fig 3-2a–b    A large discussion group with faculty and facilitator.

### 3.1    Before the course (short-term and long-term)

Appropriate case selection is very important. All members of the leading group should see and discuss the cases to be presented prior to the meeting and specific learning objectives should be agreed upon for each case. The leader of the group will determine the order of presentation. The presentation order and learning objectives should closely parallel those of the entire course. The cases should be especially clear and learning objectives should be focused in order to keep the discussion from becoming too broad. The background information presented to the audience should be brief and specific. It is often helpful to have discussion leaders prepared to discuss alternative points of view in case the audience is reluctant to participate by asking questions or giving opinions.

As stated before, the group should agree upon everyone's role. One faculty member should take the lead in presenting each case. The case leader should develop a brief presentation that includes the background of the case and the issues for discussion (preferably stated in the form of one or more questions). X-rays, slides, or other relevant visuals should be prepared (or made available in print). In preparation of the case materials consideration should be given to skill level of the course participants as well as their knowledge of the leading language.

In contrast to small discussion groups there are not many possibilities to change the layout of the lecture hall, so you have to adjust to the possibilities given. However, you should inspect the room as you would before giving a lecture, which includes lighting and AV setup. Specifically, you should know where the lighting controls are located (and how to operate them) and you should verify that the correct AV equipment is in the room and in working order. Projecting a test slide will verify that the equipment is in working order and will allow you to determine whether you will need to adjust the lighting in order for slides to be visible to the audience.

Slides or PowerPoint presentations including all the cases should be burned to disk, on CD-ROM, or memory stick and delivered to the AV technician in advance of the session. If an audience response system (ARS) is being used, someone should be stationed at the door to distribute them or they should be preplaced on each seat. Multiple wireless microphones should be available in order to make free movement of the leading group possible.

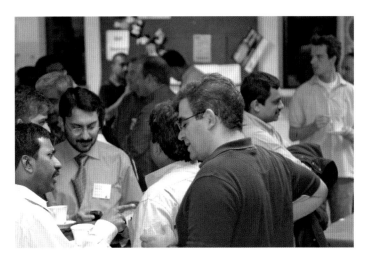

Fig 3-3    Course participants and faculty members exchanging information during informal discussions.

### 3.2    At the precourse

The material to be used in the large discussion group needs to be shown to all the faculty members at the precourse. This will allow the faculty to discuss what the learning objectives should be for any given case. It also allows the opportunity for individual faculty members to raise concerns about the suitability of the material or the correctness of the treatment modalities shown.

Since the material shown in the large discussion groups is frequently talked about by the participants during breaks, all faculty should be familiar with the material to allow them to contribute to these vital informal learning sessions **(Fig 3-3)**.

### 3.3    During the course

Like other types of presentations, a set-dialogue-closure format should be followed. The senior faculty member of the leading group should briefly introduce all members of the leading group as well as their function during this discussion group session and explain the objectives of the session and the format that will be used. The easiest way is to then let the moderator start with the first case and present the essential information for starting the discussion. Again it is important to get early participation by the course participants. There are several ways to do this. Questions, posed to the entire audience, are quick and easy ways to get the audience thinking about the case and engaged in learning. An ARS (see 1 AO education—introduction; 3 Audience response system) can be very useful in this situation because participants can respond anonymously and they can see how their responses compare to those of the rest of the group. However, use of an ARS requires preparation and a little bit of practice. Alternatives to an ARS include asking the audience to signal responses with a show of hands or to hold up colored cards indicating agreement or disagreement with a statement. Short, clear questions integrated in the slides of the case will facilitate participation of the course participants. The audience responses to questions should help the leader to determine the direction of the discussion. After some initial participation by the entire audience, the lead faculty member may ask the other faculty to make brief comments based on the responses of the audience [1].

Before asking for individual comments or questions from the audience, the other faculty should position themselves in strategic locations around the room. As the lead speaker calls on individuals, one of the faculty members should take a microphone to that individual so that the question or comment can be clearly heard by the entire audience. If wireless microphones are not available it may be possible to place one or two fixed microphones in the aisles and ask participants to come to the microphones. This method often results in a queue of several people and can help the leader judge how much time to take with each individual. Another model for eliciting participation is to allow the other faculty to move throughout the room and to choose from participants who indicate that they have a question or comment. If that method is chosen the faculty will have to move to different parts of the room to ensure wide

participation. Finally, if only one microphone is available to the lead faculty it may be necessary to require participants to shout out their question or comment to the leader. In this case the leader should remember to always repeat the question or comment to the audience before answering. It is very important that the case leader be very aware of the time.

■ ▥ **Discussion and comments should be ended after 12–15 minutes so that the main discussion leader has time to summarize the learning points of the case.**

Finally, the discussion session should end with a formal closure summing up the goals of this discussion by the lead faculty member.

### 3.3.1 Dangers and problems

Possible dangers during this session are comparable to those of the smaller discussion groups. It is not possible to have everybody make an individual comment or ask a question in a large group.

Randomly selecting members of the audience to speak can create problems by moving the discussion off target. Identifying members of the audience who are likely to have particularly useful comments or questions can be a critical variable in keeping the discussion focused on the learning objectives. Too much inconsistency or divergent opinions among the discussion leaders, although partially intended, should not turn into open controversy. Depending on the cultural backgrounds and knowledge of the leading language, the pace of the discussion may need to be adjusted.

## 3.4    After the course

A debriefing session among the faculty can be very useful for improving future discussions. Meeting informally, immediately or soon after the session, will promote a more useful discussion since the details of the session are still fresh in everyone's minds. If this is not possible, discussion leaders may agree to make evaluation notes of the session for a later discussion. The major focus of the evaluation should be on the utility of the cases selected, the ability to reach the stated learning objectives, the coordination among the faculty members, the ability to stimulate useful discussion, and the degree to which the course participants seemed to be interested and attentive to the material discussed. It is very difficult to determine the opinions of the course participants without directly asking them. If a written evaluation of the session is solicited or if other evaluation tools are used, the data should be summarized and sent to all faculty members for later discussion. If other course faculty members attended the session, it may be possible to get direct feedback and suggestions from them after the session or at a later time. Finally, any technical, environmental, or organizational issues should be discussed among the faculty.

- **Large AO discussion groups:**

  - **Are an excellent way to summarize the whole course program.**
  - **Should be guided by at least three discussion group leaders.**
  - **Need preparation in case selection and roles within leading group.**
  - **Should be presented in the set-discussion-closure format.**

## 4    Conclusion

Given the fact that the teaching/learning effects of a discussion are generally much higher than a lecture, good preparation before—and highest concentration during—these meetings are cornerstones of a successful presentation and an effective teaching moment. Faculty who show enthusiasm for teaching, an in-depth knowledge of their subject, and interest in the course participants will always have the best results in any educational setting. These characteristics create an excitement for learning that is contagious in both small and large groups.

- **The best teachers are those who are always learning their craft and are always looking for ways to improve. The suggestions described in this chapter have been shown to be successful, but all teachers must find techniques that fit their personality and style.**

## 5 Anecdote

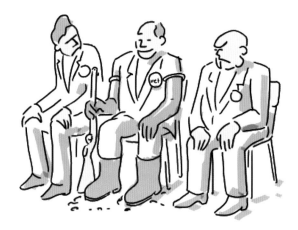

Some years ago, I had to moderate a rather large (30) "small discussion group" during an AO Principles Course. Due to a very limited time frame the introduction of the moderators was rather short, and the participants did not introduce themselves. Basic principles of fracture treatment were discussed using a case of a simple closed transverse femoral midshaft fracture in a 40-year-old farmer after being hit by a bull. The discussion was lively and many participants were involved. One participant seemed to be very interested in the case but, despite different questions, the only answers he gave were: "thank you" or "yes". After the session he unexpectedly came forward and greeted me, while asking: "what animal". I did not really understand his question and replied: "a bull, male cow". He looked amazed at me and asked: "your country?" I told him that this type of accident happens in our country and again he smiled at me and said: "Funny, we shoot them". While thinking about that answer, I was looking at his badge which clearly indicated: "Veterinary Course".

Afterwards, I learned that he indeed was a vet who had lost his group and by accident joined my small discussion group and thought that we had talked about the treatment of femoral fractures in cows.

*Roger KJ Simmermacher*

## 6    Bibliography

1. **Grasha A** (1996) *Teaching with style: A practical guide to enhancing learning by understanding learning and teaching styles.* New York: Alliance Publishers.

2. **Crosby JR, Hesketh EA** (2004) Developing the teaching instinct: Small group learning. *Medical Teacher*; 26:16–19.

3. **Walton H** (1997) Small group methods in medical teaching. *Med Ed*; 31:459–464.

4. **Jaques D** (2003) ABC of learning and teaching in medicine: Teaching small groups. *BMJ*; 326:492–494.

5. **Steinert Y** (1996) Twelve tips for effective small-group teaching in the health professions. *Medical Teacher*; 18:203–207.

Authors   Piet G de Boer, Linda Casebeer

# 4     How to run a practical

## 1     Introduction

The practical element of a course has been one of the defining characteristics of AO education from the earliest courses in the 1960s. Teaching practical skills, using cadaveric material and then plastic bone was then, 40 years ago, almost unique in the teaching of surgery. Practical exercises (practicals) remain the most widely appreciated part of an AO course when assessed by the course participants.

The use of surgical technical skill training from bench-model courses using synthetic and animal tissue or a combination of animal or cadaveric material to simulate various types of surgery has been identified as a key component in a systems approach to reducing errors in the operating theater [1]. Workshops allow hands-on demonstrations of procedures and practice, particularly suited to the teaching of surgical skills that can be learned effectively by demonstrations from experts followed by practice.

■ ⫶    **Although the most important relationship in teaching surgical skills is that between the table instructor and the course participants, the practical director has a critical role in ensuring that practicals run successfully from an educational point of view.**

The relationship between table instructors and course participants is crucial.

## 2     Before the course

### 2.1     Timing

The most common criticism of practicals is that insufficient time is given for the practical exercises. Therefore, the first task of the practical director is to establish with the course chairman that sufficient time is given within the program for the individual practical exercises.

The timing of the video is, of course, available by looking at the label on the video box, but the time required for each individual exercise can usually only be assessed by experience. If the practical director has no personal experience of the practical, discussions with colleagues and/or the chairman are vital to ensure adequate timing is given. Remember to allow time for interactivity between the table instructors and the course participants prior to starting the practical itself. Evaluations of many instructional experiences indicate that what was taught was not, in fact, learned, indicating the need for "overteaching" or repeated practice of new learnings so they can be reproduced fluently in the practice setting [2]. Also remember to allow sufficient timing for evaluation and feedback at the end of the session.

■ ⫶    **One of the most powerful effects in the instructional process is practice with feedback, and it is estimated that up to 50% of course time should be spent in practice with feedback [3, 4].**

## 2.2 Relation to the course

Practical exercises should fit naturally into the course program. The stages of mastering new skills can be summarized as:

- Acquiring knowledge of what should be done and how.
- Executing the responses in a series of steps.
- Transferring control from the eyes to other senses.
- Automatization of the skill.
- Generalization to a wider range of applications [5].

Ideally, therefore, they should be positioned after the lectures relating to the topic of the practical and adjacent to any time given for group discussion work concerning the subject matter.

The appropriate sequence is to explain **(Fig 4-1)**, demonstrate, involve, coach, and test (EDICT) [2].

### ◼▦ …explain…demonstrate…involve…coach…test

With complex exercises involving expensive course material it is not uncommon for there to be insufficient material for all the course participants to carry out the practical at the same time. Under these circumstances participants have to be divided into two groups and for the practical to take place on two separate occasions. If this is inevitable, then great care must be taken to negotiate the timetable of the practical to avoid the problem of doing a practical before the lectures relating to that topic.

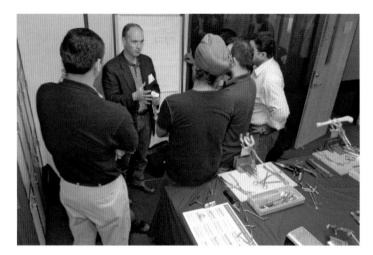

Fig 4-1    The table instructor is explaining the part of the practical after having seen the video sequence and before course participants start with the hands-on exercise.

### 2.3 Videos

The effective use of media in instruction requires an organized approach. The ASSURE model identifies various elements of this approach, including:

- Analyzing learners.
- Stating objectives.
- Selecting methods, media, and materials.
- Utilizing media and materials.
- Requiring learning outcomes.
- Evaluating the outcomes [6].

The media chosen for instruction must be able to transmit the necessary information, supply the instructional stimuli, which the content requires, and help the course participant to engage in the learning activity. For teaching practical skills, videos are the obvious choice to meet these requirements [5, 6]. However, practical aspects, such as costs and flexibility in updating the material, may influence the usefulness of any particular media [6]. Videos are usually available for each practical exercise. Videos literally take hundreds of hours to prepare and are very costly to make. Updating of videos occurs infrequently. It is important for practical directors to compare the materials' objectives against the course objectives and criteria [5].

Obtaining appropriate materials usually involves three choices:

- Finding available materials.
- Modifying existing materials.
- Designing new materials.

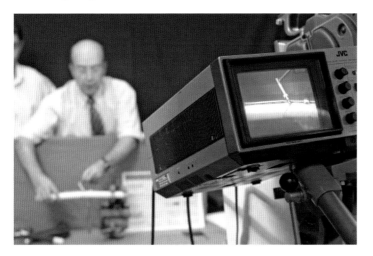

Fig 4-2    The practical director is reinforcing a critical step, previously shown in the video, by demonstrating it live over CCTV. Without preparing himself and knowing the contents of the video, he would not be able to do so.

If appropriate materials exist, time and money are saved. When materials do not match objectives, adapting materials is an option, although this is more difficult in video production than other media [6].

Most practical directors will find that the video, that has been made available for their use, does not perfectly match their teaching and learning requirements. Decisions need to be made well before the course, if this is the case. Various solutions are available:

- If there is a considerable amount of time available, it might be possible for the video studio in Davos to rework the practical video. This is expensive and time-consuming. It should therefore only be done in exceptional circumstances. In practical terms this rarely happens outside the Davos courses themselves.

- The practical director could elect to leave part of the video out, or on occasion, run part of one video and part of another one.

- The practical director might elect to do some or all of the practicals live over closed-circuit television (CCTV). This is a very high-risk strategy! Experience has shown that live demonstrations always take longer than the video themselves. Unless you have an exceptionally good cameraman and you are very experienced, the quality of the images sent over the CCTV is unlikely to match that of the teaching video available to you. For that reason, getting rid of the video is rarely advisable. Individual points which are not clear on the video can, however, be shown by a live demonstration on the CCTV (Fig 4-2).

## 2.4 Learning objectives

Most practicals now carry a list of learning objectives with them. An educational objective is a precise statement of intent of what the learner should be able to do at the end of the practical session [5]. It is critical that the practical director establishes those learning points he wishes to transmit during the practical. In choosing objectives, relevance and viability should be considered [5]. The maximum number of learning points for each individual practical is variable, but three to four would appear to be the optimum level.

■ ▥ **The practical director should carefully note his learning objectives and these should form part of his presentation to his faculty at the precourse and to the course participants during the practical itself.**

It is very useful for faculty to have a short printed handout of the learning objectives of each practical given to them at the precourse.

## 2.5 Practicals

All practicals require a certain amount of instruments and implants and an appropriate bone/soft-tissue model. Many hundreds of models now exist, and the number of teaching videos is also rapidly approaching the 100 mark. Videos have been reworked over the years to reflect changes in technique and changes in instrumentation, and it is not infrequent that a practical director would find that the video that he has been supplied, the bone model available and the instrumentation that is to be used, do not precisely match up. These problems have become considerably worse in the last 2–3 years with the introduction of LCP (locking compression plate) technologies and the rapid development of different teaching models to demonstrate this new technology. Providing the practical director finds this out sufficiently in advance, the problem can usually be resolved. Never assume that instrumentation, implants, bone model, and video will match up. Always check it with the course chairman and, if necessary, contact the industrial partner in advance.

## 2.6 Chunking

The videos provided vary in length from 5–25 minutes. Traditionally, AO practicals involved running the video from start to finish and then allowing the course participants to proceed with the exercise. It is clearly impossible for the course participants to fully appreciate the entire length of a complex practical and, therefore, practical directors must, before the course, decide how they are going to divide the practical up into manageable (learnable) "chunks". The traditional approach of presenting lengthy sets of content proves less than optimal as a teaching tool. The "chunked" method, on the other hand, is an excellent format for formal small and large-group instruction [7]. The most frequent error in instructional design is to make the chunks of instruction too large [4]. Once the nature of the chunks has been established, practical directors should then decide which other key steps are involved and what the learning objectives of each section of the practical should be.

■ ▥ **Careful planning and timing of the individual chunks is essential for digestible learning portions.**

Once this has been done, a timetable for the running of the practical can be constructed. This timetable would include the start time and the time that the practical director feels would be necessary for each particular chunk of the practical to take place. Included into the timetable would be the learning objectives of the practical as a whole and the key points for each particular section or chunk of the practical. This document can form the basis of a handout at the precourse as well as an aide memoire for the director himself while the practical is running.

Future AO teaching DVDs will be prechunked with information available as to the length of each particular chunk.

## 2.7    Venue and setup

The setup for most practicals include TVs within the practical room to allow the course participants to see the video. Most practicals have a CCTV system so that the practical director can appear on these TV screens. The quality of the camera work varies enormously from venue to venue. Some long-established courses have professional cameramen and sound technicians managing the CCTV. Most courses have a hand-held, or tripod-mounted camcorder with limited zooming facilities. The practical director must check, in advance, what is available for his particular practical and talk with the cameraman/technician to tell him exactly what is required during the practical. It is useful to be able to project onto the TV screens the aims and objectives of the practicals as well as the key points for each chunk of it. This can be done through a camcorder focused on a flip chart (**Fig 4-3**). Other alternatives include the use of a computer and projector.

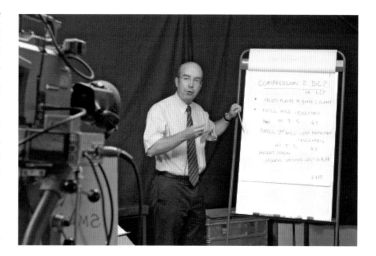

Fig 4-3    Camcorder focused on flip chart and practical director. It is important that the practical director checks the equipment and discusses the requirements with the technician in advance.

## 2.8    Preparing your presentation

As with formal lectures, an important part of the instructional design process is to start by defining your conclusions. This is the most important part of your message and the one that is most likely to be remembered by the course participants [4, 5]. Clearly your conclusions should be based on the learning points that you wish to bring out throughout the presentation. Then work backwards through the presentation, thinking about the learning objectives for each particular section of the practical and finally prepare the introduction.

## 3     At the precourse

The amount of work that you have to do at the precourse will depend largely on the faculty that you have been allocated to help you with the practical. In rare incidences, all the faculty members will already be familiar with the practical and with the learning objectives from it. Most of the time, however, your faculty will vary from those who are extremely experienced to those who are just starting their AO teaching career as a table instructor.

### 3.1     Learning objectives

The key to success of the practical is to ensure that the table instructors providing the one-on-one teaching and learning experience are familiar and content with the learning objectives that you have decided are important for a given practical. In most incidences no problems will arise—but on occasion some faculty members (usually senior) may have other ideas about what the nature of the learning objectives are for a particular practical. Their concerns must be discussed openly at the precourse and a common line agreed upon. A key to effective instructional design, which leads to desired outcomes, is consensus on the desired outcomes as stated in the learning objectives that are communicated to learners [4].

■ ▦     **Key is to:**

- ▦ **Decide on learning objectives.**
- ▦ **Agree on learning objectives with faculty at precourse.**
- ▦ **Communicate learning objectives to course participants.**

### 3.2     Timetable

The precourse is the opportunity for you, as the practical director, to produce the timetable for the practical. This will give the table instructors an understanding of the time constraints under which they are operating and how the practical is to be split up.

### 3.3     Video

Traditionally, the practical videos have been played at the precourse in their entirety. This has, in the past, led to very long, tedious, and unpopular precourses, and it is unreasonable to expect faculty members to watch upwards of 3 hours of video, while maintaining even the slightest degree of interest. It is therefore best to only use videos for controversial or difficult points. Most course chairmen now circulate the videos to be used in the practicals to all the relevant faculty members before the course. This is usually in a CD-ROM format. Note that although CD-ROMs can be used on your laptop to prepare for courses, they do not give sufficient clarity of image to be used on the courses themselves. A DVD-video format will be available in 2005 to get around this problem. In theory, therefore, all the relevant faculty members will have had an opportunity to review the videos before the course begins. Do not, however, make that assumption. The vast majority of faculty members do not preview the videos until shortly before the practical, and it is unwise to assume a familiarity of the material while discussing it at the precourse.

## 3.4    Deviation

Nearly all of the faculty will be considerably more senior than the course participants. They are usually fairly experienced surgeons and—like most orthopedic surgeons—have developed their own particular ways of performing an operation. The teaching videos used in a practical represent best practice; but most if not all, of the faculty will have in the course of their career, developed various tricks and tips when dealing with a particular clinical problem. There is an overwhelming desire on the part of the table instructors to confer this additional knowledge to the course participants. How often have you heard "I know that they do it this way in the video, but if I were you, I would just do it this way". To the individual practitioner such advice may seem, at best, highly useful and at worst, harmless; but the reality is that if the faculty covertly or overtly disagree with the teaching video then the confidence of the course participants is severely dented. It is therefore wise at the precourse to ask all the faculty members present if there are any aspects of the practical with which they disagree and have an open discussion as to what the common approach is going to be. Faculty must understand that it is better for them to take a united stand, advocating one particular line of therapy even if individual members of the faculty believe that there maybe better ways of doing things.

■ ▥    **Faculty must understand that it is better for them to take a united stand, advocating one particular line of therapy even if individual members of the faculty believe that there maybe better ways of doing things.**

## 3.5    Running the precourse session

The precourse or shortly afterwards is the last time that the practical instructor has to ensure that the appropriate teaching material is available. The effective use of media and materials, as defined by the ASSURE, requires previewing the materials and making sure all media and materials are available and fit the required teaching scenario [6]. It is also his opportunity to check out the AV system, the CCTV, and to discuss with the cameraman/technician exactly how he wishes to proceed and how he wishes the video to be divided up and shown.

Most AO courses extend between 3 and 5 days. For 4- and 5-day courses it is probably wise to not discuss all the practicals at the precourse, but to discuss the first ones at the precourse and the subsequent ones at the faculty meetings that are held regularly throughout the course.

## 4    During the course

### 4.1    Setup

Always arrive 10–15 minutes before the session is due to start and ensure that your teaching material is correct. This is also an opportunity for you to have last-minute discussions with the cameraman and technician with regard to how you wish him to cooperate during the course. If you are doing the first practical of a course then go into the practical room to check out the visibility of the screens and the audibility of the sound system.

### 4.2    Introductions

Introductions should be brief and to the point. They should include the learning objectives of the practicals.

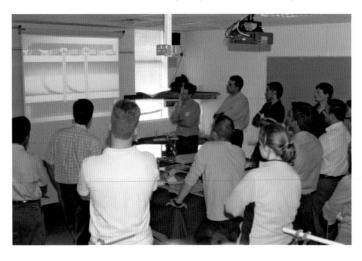

Fig 4-4    It is important, that course participants fully concentrate on the video chunk. The hands-on work must therefore stop immediately as soon as the television screen comes on.

Trying to put a degree of clinical relevance into it is also a very good attention grabber. The introduction serves as an advance organizer and an aid to effective instruction; an advance organizer may include an overview of the information, a statement of principles contained in the information, and a statement of objectives. Studies have demonstrated the contribution of an advance organizer to the increased effectiveness of instructional courses [6, 8]. The introduction is also an opportunity for the practical director to inform the course participants how he wishes the practical to run. If you are conducting the first practical then information also needs to be given with regard to safety, goggles, sharps, etc. It is also essential for the practical director of the first practical to inform the course participants that following cessation of the video he will expect them to link up with their table instructor for a brief discussion before commencing work on the practical. Finally, mention must of course be made that when the television screens come on, all work should cease promptly **(Fig 4-4)**.

### 4.3    Handing over to the table instructors

The course participants, having heard the introduction and watched the first part of the video, will be incredibly keen to start working immediately. It is therefore vital that when the video stops, the practical director comes back onto the CCTV screen to direct the course participants to their table instructors and to lay out the nature of the discussion that he wishes them to have. A useful way of ensuring that course participants do not start the practical too early is to ensure that the air supply for the power tools is not switched on immediately after the video stops. This requires careful negotiations with the technical staff who naturally prefer to have the air switched on for the whole of the session.

## 4.4    Timing

The practical director must keep a close eye on the timing throughout the practical. If a table instructor brings to his attention the fact that many of the course participants are making the same mistake, then it is worth pointing that out to the course participants before the next set of videos are shown. Be very careful, however, at showing course participants work on the CCTV. Course participants do not take kindly to public humiliation. Having their genuine mistakes put on public display provides a very negative form of feedback to them.

Most practical directors do stroll around the room during the practical, to get a sense of how things are working.

■ ▦ **On occasion timing goes badly array. If it is clear that a practical is going to overrun then two options are available:**

▦ **The practical can be allowed to continue for the appropriate required length. You can really only do this if you are talking about 10 minutes or so, because the 10 minutes extra, that your practical takes up, will inevitably eat into 10 minutes of free time available to the course participants. All courses are extremely intense experiences for faculty and participants alike. Both faculty and participants require some down time during the day to reflect on what they have seen and learned and to allow them some time to recharge their intellectual batteries. Also remember that coffee breaks often provide the best informal learning conditions on any course.**

▦ **Cut out the last sections of the practicals. It is far better to do three-quarters of a practical correctly than to rush through the whole practical in an effort to meet a time deadline. There is a natural tendency on behalf of faculty and course participants alike to feel that the most important thing in a practical session is to complete the exercise. Although this is important, rushing through rarely produces good learning outcomes.**

## 4.5    Discipline

Discipline can be very hard to maintain during courses. There is considerable variation worldwide as to what is and what is not acceptable behavior amongst the course participants. In many parts of the world and in many courses, course participants do not stop work when the television screens come on. Ignoring this never works and even though it may take a minute or so to restore order, this is time that is very well worth taking.

## 4.6    Summarize

At the end of the practical, summarize the learning objectives for the course [4]. Try to concentrate on the positive aspects of the work that has been shown and don't dwell on any problems that arose. Ensure that the course participants leave the room with a clear understanding of what was required of them and what they have done and give clear directions as to their next assignments.

## 5 After the course

### 5.1 Chairman's report

Techniques change, videos alter, and equipment becomes more or less complex. Therefore, some practicals that used to be rushed through in one hour, can now be comfortably handled in 3/4 hour. Other practicals have grown in their complexity and time requirements. New videos, which have been meticulously worked out, may on their first time of showing turn out to contain serious potential errors and areas of ambiguity. New bone models, which worked perfectly in testing, may fracture with monotonous regularity in a course situation.

Feedback is therefore essential to give your successor some idea of the successes and failures of your practical and the potential pitfalls to avoid. This serves as a means of formative evaluation, allowing for important revisions when the course is next offered [5]. If any issues therefore do arise, you are advised to communicate with the course chairman, so that appropriate modification can be made in subsequent courses.

### 5.2 Participant assessment

At present, the AO carries out no formal long-term assessment of the effect that skills' training has in the surgical practice of the course participants. Experience at the courses has shown us that most participants can have the psychomotor skills improved considerably as a result of the experience of going through an AO practical. We do not know, however, whether this experience is translated into their everyday practice after the course.

### 5.3 Conclusion

Practicals remain one of the bedrocks of AO education. The success or failure of the learning experience will be largely determined by interaction between the table instructors and the course participants. It is the job of the practical director to structure the learning experience in such a way that this relationship can be optimized. Meticulous plan of the practical before the course, together with the creation of agreed learning objectives and a timetable, are the keys to success. The days of run the video and now do the practical are over.

## 6    Anecdote

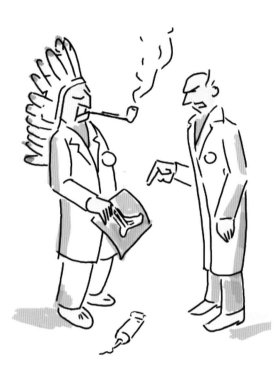

*Even the most experienced educators, in the end, meet their match. Full of confidence I was asked to sort out a problem during a practical in Davos. What had happened was that six of the course participants had decided to fix the ankle fracture in an extremely idiosyncratic way, bearing no relationship at all to what the video had suggested. The table instructor had said that he had been unable to resolve the issue and I approached the table, brimming full of confidence. Standing with an open stance—and in the friendliest possible way—I enquired in the correct fashion "My, that looks very interesting, can you tell me why you do it this way?" There was a brief pause, and the course participants replied together "Because that is the way we do things in our hospital". Not put off, I then asked "Can you tell me why you do it this way in your hospital?" Quick as a flash came the answer, "Because our professor tells us to do it this way". I still was not beaten, so asked "But can you tell me why your professor asks you to do it in this particular way". There was a brief pause, and the answer came back "Because that is the way we do it in our hospital". After two more circuits round this somewhat curious conversation, I gave up. Modern AO teaching techniques cannot cope with hierarchical medical systems that have been in use for many centuries.*

*Piet G de Boer*

## 7    Bibliography

1.  **Sudip SK** (2003) Courses, cadavers, and counsellors: reducing errors in the operating theatre. *BMJ*; 327:109.
2.  **Farquharson A** (1995) *Teaching in practice.* San Francisco: Jossey-Bass Publishers.
3.  **Branch RM, Kent L** (1997) *Survey of instructional development models.* 3rd ed. Syracuse, New York: Information Resource Publications.
4.  **Dick WO, Carey L, Carey JO** (2000) *The systematic design of instruction.* 5th ed. Upper Saddle River, New Jersey: Pearson, Allyn & Bacon.
5.  **Romiszkowski AJ** (1999) *Designing instructional systems.* 2nd ed. New York: Nichols Publishing.
6.  **Heinich R, Molenda M, Russell JD, et al** (1999) *Instructional media and technologies for learning.* 6th ed. Upper Saddle River, New Jersey: Merrill.
7.  **Brose JA** (1992) Case presentation as a teaching tool: making a good thing better. *J Am Osteopath Assoc.* Mar; 92(3):376–8.
8.  **Ausubel D, Novak J, Hanesian H** (1978) *Educational Psychology: A Cognitive View.* 2nd ed. New York: Holat, Rinehart & Winston.

Authors    Ian Harris, Robert D Fox

# 5    How to be a table instructor

## 1    Introduction

Although the knowledge gained from lectures and discussions underpin the development of skills needed in the operating room, it is the hands-on experience with the equipment that results in success.

■ ▦    **The table instructor serves as coach, mentor, and facilitator of learning as course participants strive to master the processes and tools of surgery.**
**He is the first line of contact for the course participants during the practical demonstrations.**

It is unlikely that any course participant would be able to perform and understand the practical exercises (practicals) with only the video demonstration and supervisor's comments. It is the table instructor's role to see that the participant understands the concepts and is able to perform the tasks that are put forward, and that they carry that knowledge with them back to the operating room.

The role of the table instructor is to supervise activity at one table during practical demonstrations. A table will usually have between four and eight participants and, if the number is large and manpower allows, there may be two table instructors per table. The table instructor is usually a surgeon with some experience using the equipment and techniques being demonstrated. The techniques will vary depending on the type of course.

The central value of the table instruction is the opportunity it presents for learners to integrate experience with cognition. Adult learners depend on experience for learning; experiences they have had in the past and experiences they have while learning in the present [1, 2]. The ability to remember and apply what was learned at the program depends on the extent to which the information can be associated with past experiences—and therefore dependably stored in the memory—and the extent to which it can be translated reliably into practice behavior.

■ ▦    **It is the experience at the table, coaching by the table instructor, and reflective interaction that characterizes this kind of the learning experience that transforms learning into actions at the point of care.**

The practical demonstrations and attempts at practice are important parts of any course. They require careful planning and good communication and coordination between the practical director and the table instructors, and good communication between the table instructors and the course participants.

Just as experience with the processes, techniques, and equipment allow course participants to store and recall information from their long-term memory, interaction and feedback at the table assure better practices upon return to their regular practices [3]. Interaction allows the course participants to see the interrelationship between actions and interpret and evaluate their performance based on feedback [4]. Interaction—particularly among participants—also provides emotional support during the trial and error needed to refine skills. Finally, interaction provides for self-assessment of knowledge and skills so that limits are identified and future self-directed learning is guided and directed. Clearly, learning will be facilitated more effectively with targeted and constructive interaction of course participants among themselves and with the table instructor.

This chapter will cover the responsibilities of the table instructor before, during, and after the course. Interspersed are explanations as to why this is important and how it affects learning and change.

At the conclusion of this chapter, the reader should be able to:

- Facilitate learning of critical concepts and surgical skills by participants.
- Supervise the hands-on instruction provided during the practical exercises with the equipment.
- Link current learning objectives to learners' past experiences to facilitate remembering of concepts and skills.
- Assist learners to be able to apply what they learn back to their practice environment.
- Facilitate interaction among learners and between faculty and participants.
- Assist learners to set goals for future self-directed learning efforts.

## 2    Before the course

The main tasks of the table instructor before the course are directed towards:

- Familiarization.
- Growing comfortable with the process.
- Preparing for the teaching/learning transaction.

One should be familiar with the surgical equipment and procedures of the practical, but also with the video presentation and supervisors' plans for the practical.

### 2.1    Familiarization with the surgical procedures

It is likely that you will be familiar with the type of procedures being demonstrated, eg, femoral nailing, but it will be helpful if you examined your own technique before getting to the course. Many people can perform intramedullary nailing with little effort (and hopefully good results) but may not be conscious of each step they are taking and will, therefore, not be able to communicate that to others. This is because your knowledge may be tacit, known to you in a way that allows you to use it but not known explicitly. Schön [5] refers to this as knowledge and skills that are embedded in actions rather than consciously thought through.

■ ■    **The challenge of the expert table instructor is to make their implicit knowledge explicit so that it can be transmitted to course participants.**

Also, many surgeons pick up various habits along the way that may or may not be useful. Depending on your equipment and facilities, you may have adapted previously taught techniques over time. These techniques may vary from that being taught in the practical, and may in fact be poor techniques. Regardless of their usefulness, introducing them to participants who are unfamiliar with the basic principles of the procedure may be harmful or even contradictory to the technique being demonstrated. At best, they may confuse the participant.

■ ▥    **Making tacit knowledge and skills explicit allows for examination, reflection, and refinements before you attempt to transmit them to the course participants at your table.**

The best way to grow familiar with the techniques being demonstrated at the table is to refer to the AO textbook covering the topic, eg, the "AO Principles of Fracture Management". Use this to self-audit and self-correct before you face course participants at your table. The video to be used during the practical should also be viewed prior to the course. This may be difficult if they are not at hand. In North America videos can be viewed through the eRoom system. In many countries CD-ROMs of the practical exercises are distributed to faculty members with the precourse material. If you have difficulty in obtaining a video you can contact AO International or the local representative of the industrial partner. At present, the Internet is a variable resource: watching streamed videos is time consuming and the presence of firewalls often makes it impossible. The opening of the AO portal in 2005 may improve this situation.

## 2.2    Familiarization with the surgical equipment

The equipment and implants used at your institution may differ from those used in the practicals. You may use a completely different system or a different version of the same system. If you usually use a different system from the one being demonstrated, you will need to view and lay your hands on the right equipment. If it is not available at your institution, your local AO or industrial partner representative should be able to arrange for you to spend some time familiarizing yourself with the equipment.

If you are using the same equipment, it is likely that the equipment used during the demonstrations will vary in some way. This is due to updates in some equipment, as well as international variations. The equipment should match that seen in the instructional video, but to be on the safe side, this should be confirmed.

## 2.3    Connection with the course chairman

The course program will usually undergo several revisions before being finalized. You should make sure that you have the final version of the course program and check the topics, dates, times, and directors of the practicals to which you are assigned. Also take note of any communication from the course chairman. The educational work that happens at the table is part of an overall plan. Knowledge of that plan can help you foster the integration of learning from other venues with the practice you are facilitating at the table. When planning your travel, make sure that you arrive in time for the precourse meeting.

## 3　At the precourse

All of the faculty members (including practical directors and table instructors) should be at the precourse meeting. It is helpful to get acquainted with members of the faculty and other demonstrators. This will make any discussion necessary during the course much easier.

During the precourse meeting, each practical exercise will be discussed and the practical director will outline the learning objectives and the timetable for the practicals. If you are not provided with a handout of the practical outlines, then you should take notes during the discussion.

Preview the workstations and find out how many participants and table instructors will be at each table. You can also get an idea of how much room there will be, what your view of the video will be, and where the practical director will be based.

If you have not already done so, it may be helpful to preview the videos at this time but time will be limited, and this is best done prior to arriving at the course. You may also be able to preview the instruments, bones, and implants that will be used.

## 4　During the course

### 4.1　Get to know the participants at your table

Before the practical commences there are usually a few minutes, when the course participants are at the table before the session starts. This is the time to start to get to know them. You are their first point of contact throughout the practical exercises and familiarization will improve communication at the table and also make the process more enjoyable for you and the participants. Introductions and name tags are useful. Asking questions about their background as well as allowing them to talk will also make it easier for them to ask questions later, and it will provide you with valuable information regarding their level of knowledge and experience with the techniques being taught.

One of the most useful outcomes of preliminary contact is to allow for an informal needs assessment. This is especially important since needs and motivation are intertwined [6].

■ ▪ **Learning needs may be thought of as the discrepancy between what is and what ought to be. This discrepancy creates a sense of unease when it is large enough. The unease, essentially a low-grade anxiety, generates a drive to reduce the discrepancy between what is and what ought to be. Although this discrepancy may be real or perceived, it is the perception of the discrepancy that charges motivation.**

Thus, if you can identify and assist the course participants to identify areas of discrepancy between what is and what ought to be, you can increase their attention and motivation to learn essential knowledge and skills. On the other hand, if you identify areas where they experience little discrepancy between where they are and where they ought to be, these areas may not receive the attention they may deserve. This is particularly important when their perception that they are where they ought to be is incorrect or their perception of where they are is incorrect.

■  ⅲ    **The feedback and interaction you foster at the table can correct misperceptions and cause the unmotivated to become motivated to learn [7].**

Not only will interaction with course participants make it easier for them to ask questions and for you to teach them, but they will be more likely to ask questions if they are comfortable with you. Many participants at courses feel overwhelmed or embarrassed and will not ask questions. This limits their understanding of the topic and makes the experience less satisfying. You can foster openness among course participants by not only getting to know them, but also showing them you are approachable. Comments such as "There is no such thing as a stupid question", or "If there are any points that you don't understand, please put up your hand straight away and let me know" will make it more comfortable for them to ask questions.

Adults are oriented to problems and are self-directed by nature. Most of what physicians learn reflects this orientation to independence and preference for learning around practical problems rather than concepts [8]. Engage your course participants on this basis, and they will not only increase their knowledge retention but also enhance their sensation of the "AO spirit".

## 4.2    Reinforce the demonstration

The practicals are usually run in segments. For example, a 12-minute video on intramedullary nailing may be broken up into five segments (chunks): entry point creation and guide wire insertion, reaming, nail insertion, nail locking, and nail extraction. After each segment of the video, the practical director may add some comments before the participants start. It is useful for the table instructor to spend 1 or 2 minutes going over what the course participants are to do during that segment, to reinforce the steps and to ensure that each of the steps and the principles involved are understood **(Fig 5-1)**. This is best done at the beginning, because once the air-powered drills start, communication is usually limited to surgeon pairs, rather than the whole table, due to the noise of the drills.

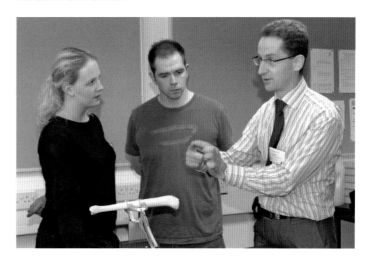

Fig 5-1    It is of utmost importance that the table instructor explains the steps shown in the video and discuss the principles involved before the course participants start with the hands-on exercise.

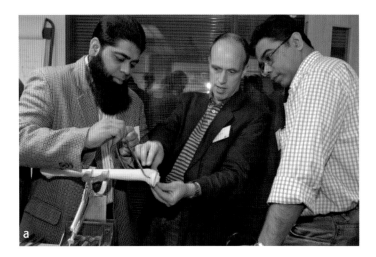 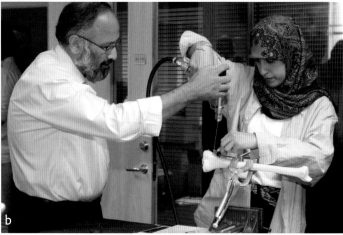

Fig 5-2a–b   Controlled supervision during the exercise is important—but do not step in too early, let the course participants discover their own mistakes. Coach them in a way that they are able to retrieve the stored knowledge and skill later in their operating room.

## 4.3    Controlled supervision

Schön [5] encourages teachers to act as coaches, encouraging learners to gain experience while being prepared to direct their reflective processes as they learn. Once the course participants begin, watch for any technical errors or any participants who cannot proceed and may need help. However, you must avoid the temptation to step in too early and do the exercise for them, or to quickly tell them the correct way and then move on. It is very helpful for the course participants to discover their own mistakes, so comments such as "Where do you think you may have gone wrong here?" or "How could you have done that differently?" may be used. Allow them to "discover" the right way of doing things as much as possible as this will provide better retention **(Fig 5-2)**.

## ■ ▥    Practice is a fundamental principle of learning.

Practice is a fundamental principle of learning. It is essential to memory. You are teaching a skill that must be stored in memory so your ability to make the most of the practice time at the table is critical to success. Remember that learning is cyclical and interactive. Kolb [9] described learning as a dialectical process moving from having a "concrete experience" drawing "reflective observations" about the experience, making an "abstract conceptualization" for storing and retrieving information, and active experimentation with the new competency. Coach them with this cycle in mind. Interact with them in a way that helps them to store this knowledge and skill for retrieval later, in their own operating theater.

## 4.4   Maintain control over the timing

The practical exercises need to run to a tight schedule (**Fig 5-3**). This will be partly the responsibility of the practical director, but for each segment, you will need to make sure your group is able to complete their tasks on time. Don't spend too long talking to them, and if they are too slow, you may need to help them through some of the time-consuming steps so that they are prepared for the next segment.

Conversely, don't let any of the course participants go too far ahead. It is usual for some of the surgeons to be faster than the others, but if one pair goes too far ahead, they may find that they have used an incorrect technique. In any case, it may cause frustration amongst the slower surgeons.

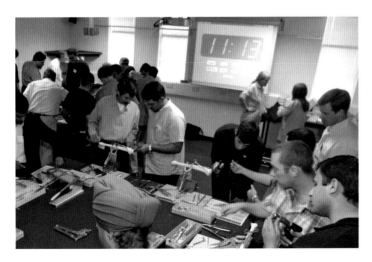

Fig 5-3   In order to keep time control, it is very helpful to have the running time displayed on screen during the exercise.

## 4.5   Ensure participant comprehension

Participants may find themselves mimicking the procedures on the video and end up with a good result, but will not understand the concepts behind the procedure. This can be elaborated during the group discussion between presentation of the video and the hands-on for each segment, but, if in doubt, a question like "Do you understand why we did it this way?" may be quite revealing. As mentioned earlier, guided reflection about their experience is an excellent way to help them get it right and understand why [10].

There is often a break at the end of each practical, so the course participants should be asked if they understood the session or if they have any questions at the end of the session. They may feel more comfortable asking questions (and you may feel more comfortable answering them) without the pressure of time constraints that exist during the practical exercise. This is the part of learning from experience Schön [5] refers to as "reflection on actions". It is essential to incorporating the new competencies into their patterns of practice.

## 4.6   Stick to the script

It may be tempting to "show off" your knowledge about a particular technique by demonstrating alternative techniques, which you may use. Although the intention may be to increase the knowledge of the participants, the effect may be otherwise. In fact, this kind of approach may result in the alternative knowledge interfering with the primary knowledge and skill the session is designed to foster [3]. The techniques described have been carefully designed to allow the course participants to retain them and reproduce them without error, adding alternatives to the recognized techniques may confuse the surgeons, if not at the time, then later when they try to reproduce them at their own institution.

### 4.7    Feedback to course participants

At the end of each session, it is useful to provide some feedback to each of the surgeons. It is helpful for them to know that they have completed the practical satisfactorily. Your comments should always be supportive, even if you wish to highlight some areas of weakness. An appropriate comment might be "You did that exercise well, but don't forget to countersink interfragmentary screws that do not lie in a plate".

■■    **Feedback is essential in all learning situations because it allows course participants to edit and correct the knowledge and skill, making their memory and their performance better. Physicians want feedback on their performance and they will see this as an excellent opportunity to get it.**

However, remember that feedback given poorly is not helpful to learning [4]. Consider their feelings of vulnerability given the public nature of the learning experience and the presence of peers. Also, remember that you want them to be "self-correcting" in their surgical practices so feedback should not only guide, but also explain.

### 4.8    Keep an eye on the rest of the practical: problems and how to deal with them

It is helpful to see how other groups are proceeding. It may give you some idea of how to pace the practical, and you often see the same mistake occurring at several tables, which you may want to bring to the attention of your group. In the following the most common problems during a course are described and solutions offered.

### 4.8.1    Nonattendance of course participants

The practical exercises are an important part of the course and certification of course completion or CME credit cannot be given if a course participant does not attend the practical exercises. You should have a list of which participants are expected to be at your table and if there is a course participant absent you should attempt to contact them and let the course chairman know.

Some participants may feel that the practicals are unnecessary. If this is the case, the importance of the sessions should be explained to them, and it should be pointed out that even experienced surgeons can gain a lot from the practical exercise.

If a course participant refuses to attend the practical exercise, then the matter should be handled by the course chairman.

### 4.8.2    Lack of experience with certain procedures or implants

If you are unfamiliar with the procedure being demonstrated the course participants will know. It will diminish their learning for that procedure and they will have a lack of confidence in your ability for the other practicals. It is better to be honest in these situations and say that you are unfamiliar with that particular technique. Working off the video, or asking a fellow instructor will usually ensure that teaching is not interrupted.

### 4.8.3   Participants with poor understanding

Occasionally, a course participant will have persistent difficulty understanding the topics discussed, despite explanation. This is most commonly due to language difficulties. It may be helpful in these cases to explain the concept at a slower pace at the end of the practical exercise. Enlisting the help of a fellow countryman with better language skills may also help.

### 4.8.4   When there is more than one instructor

When there is more than one table instructor per table, the instructors should decide how they are to manage the group before the first practical. It is usually easier to divide the table in two, with each instructor having their own group, but each continuing to be available to the others if required.

### 4.8.5   Course participants going too far ahead

Timing is difficult in practical exercises but occasionally some surgeons will race ahead of the others, especially if they have some familiarity with the techniques. It should be suggested that they do not go on to the next segment before it is presented, as they will understand the procedure better if they perform it after it has been explained. If they complete their tasks early, ask them to observe a colleague and be prepared to provide feedback if requested by the instructor.

### 4.8.6   Spending too long with one course participant

Instructors should be careful not to spend much of their time on a particularly slow or demanding course participant to the detriment of the other surgeons. If a participant requires more supervision than usual, you may need to spend time with them at the end of the session.

## 5    After the course

After the course, feedback to others involved in the planning and instructional processes of the course may be useful. You may wish to give feedback to the course chairman and practical director regarding aspects of the practical exercises that went well or could be improved such as particularly difficult sections, timing or equipment problems. You should also ask the practical director for feedback, they will usually be patrolling the floor during the practical exercises and may have some advice for you.

The most important feedback may come from the course participants. It is helpful to ask them if they thought the practical exercise went well, or if they had any comments regarding any aspects of the practicals, not only regarding your performance, but any general points, which you may want to pass on to the practical director and course chairman.

## 6 Summary of principles of effective coaching for table instructors

Working as a table instructor will be effective if you stay close to some fundamental principles of this kind of teaching and learning.

- The most important part of the course is the direct experience of the course participants. It is the basis for incorporating all knowledge and skill into real-life surgical practices.

- You are a coach as they attempt to master the knowledge and skills. You need to be trusted in this role for not only your competence as a surgeon, but also your competence as a person. You are a role model for the course participants, and it is in this way that you can change their attitudes and their skills.

- Interaction is the key to storing this knowledge and skill in the memory in a way that is retrievable when they are "back home". Interaction helps the course participant to associate this experience with existing competencies and practices. It is fine-tuning but also intellectual practice at storing and retrieving what is needed to perform successfully.

- Your knowledge is tacit, embedded in your actions. You must make your knowledge explicit, visible to the learner, so that they can understand it, practice it, and store it.

- Motivation is driven by the ability of course participants to compare present knowledge and skills with required knowledge and skills. Your ability to give feedback in a way that enables course participants to see where they are and where they ought to be is fundamental to enhancing motivation to learn.

- Like most adult learners, these surgeons are independent, practical, and problem-oriented in their approach to learning. However they must also be reflective. They must know why, not just how. Coaching means directing, correcting, and explaining.

The role of the table instructor is central to success for this program. It is a point of integration and the basis for reflection for the other components of the course. It depends on your surgical, educational, and interpersonal knowledge and skill. Be transparent in what you do and teach them in a way that makes them want to learn.

## 7    Anecdote

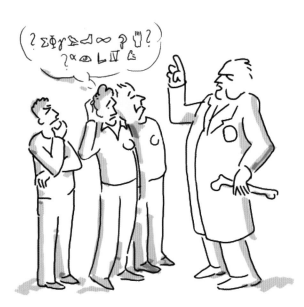

*During a basic course that involved international participants, I was table instructor to surgeons from several different countries. One participant did not have good conversational English skills but seemed to understand most of the instructions I gave. It was not until near the end of the first practical exercise, that I realized he had not understood the points I had made and was not able to understand the video. He had been nodding when I explained things to him, but only out of politeness, not because he understood what I was saying. The same thing has happened with patients who have perfect language skills but do not understand the concepts being explained: often course participants will not wish to appear obstructive, impolite, or lacking in knowledge. It is important that you confirm the course participants understanding of each topic—perhaps by asking them to tell you what their understanding of the subject is.*

*Ian Harris*

## 8    Bibliography

1. **Knowles MS** (1984) *The Adult Learner: A Neglected Species.* 3rd ed. Houston: Gulf.
2. **Merriam SB, Caffarella RS** (1999) *Learning in Adulthood: A Comprehensive Guide.* 2nd ed. San Francisco: Jossey-Bass.
3. **Gagne RM, Briggs LJ, Wager WW** (1992) *Principles of Instructional Design.* 4th ed. Orlando: Harcourt Brace.
4. **Bennett NL, Fox RD** (2003) Feedback and Reminder Systems. *Davis DA, Barnes BE, Fox RD (eds). The Continuing Professional Development of Physicians: From Theory to Practice.* Chicago: AMA Press.
5. **Schön DA** (1990) *Educating the reflective practitioner: toward a new design for teaching and learning in the professions.* San Francisco: Jossey-Bass Publishers.
6. **Fox RD, Bennett NL** (1998) Learning and change: implications for continuing medical education. *BMJ*; 316(7129):466–468.
7. **Fox RD, Miner C** (1999) Motivation and the Facilitation of Change, Learning and Participation in Educational Programs for Health Professionals. *Journal of Continuing Education in the Health Professions;* 19(3).
8. **Mann KV, Gelula MH** (2003) How to facilitate self-directed learning. *Davis DA, Barnes BE, Fox RD (eds). The Continuing Professional Development of Physicians: From Theory to Practice.* Chicago: AMA Press
9. **Kolb DA** (1984) *Experiential learning: Experience as the source of learning and development.* Englewood Cliffs: Prentice Hall.
10. **Fox RD, Craig J** (1994) Future Directions for Research on Physicians as Learners. *Davis DA, Fox RD (eds). The physician as learner: Linking research to practice.* Chicago: AMA Press.

Authors  KokSun Khong, Lisa Hadfield-Law

# 6  How to give a lecture

## 1  Introduction

A great lecture rarely comes about by chance. It is not uncommon when beginning to develop an outline of a lecture to find yourself trying to cram in everything you know about a topic—citing references galore, showcasing your most exciting cases, and then squeezing all this into a 20-minute lecture. For those who are reasonably proficient in the use of PowerPoint, you then proceed to fill every slide with as much information as you can, and produce a 70-slide lecture, often with fancy backgrounds, font style, and colors. You might polish this off with moving graphics or even sound effects, in an attempt to use everything the program can provide. Disappointment prevails when participants whisper, complain that you overran, or give the perfunctory clap... or sigh of relief. More importantly perhaps, the opportunity to contribute to learning is lost.

This chapter is designed to help you give an effective lecture on an AO course. The educational principles underpinning the suggestions are integrated into the main text so that you will understand the theory of what you are doing. Much of the research into the effectiveness of lectures was conducted some years ago, which perhaps reflects the focus of educational research today. By the end of this chapter the reader will be able to:

- Prepare a lecture to be delivered at an AO course.
- Select a suitable method of delivery.
- Use technology effectively.
- Consider how to manage special circumstances, eg, overrunning your allotted time, different cultures, hostility, and technical problems.

## 1.1  Aim of the lecture

- Provide useful and clinically applicable information.
- Introduce concepts or ideas which will be developed through discussion and practical exercises (practicals).
- Include information which is up-to-date and evidence-based.
- Make sure course participants have the same baseline knowledge.
- Motivate course participants to want to learn more.

## 1.2  Limitation of lectures

A lecture is a valuable learning tool when linked with sufficient opportunities for course participants to reflect, process, and apply what they have learned from a lecture, for example, discussions and practical skills exercises. Smeltzer et al [1] showed that learners listen more closely if they know there is going to be a discussion on what the lecturer is saying.

■ ▥  **After the introduction, remind the audience that they will require the knowledge you are about to deliver for a practical exercise or case discussion, for example, preoperative planning steps, dynamic compression plating for stable fixation, or decision-making in a polytrauma patient.**

However, despite all the characteristics of an effective presentation, mounting evidence shows that the traditional teacher-dominated lecture is inadequate for facilitating higher-level learning and behavioral change [2–4].

■ ▦ ▨ **Bligh [5] combines decades of experience as a faculty developer and in-depth knowledge of the research literature, to draw the conclusion that lectures should be used to teach information. They should not be relied upon to promote thought, change attitudes, or develop behavioral skills.**

Lectures, however, remain an important component of AO courses so you will need to develop the appropriate skills and characteristics of a good lecturer.

## 1.3 The effective lecturer

- Demonstrates enthusiasm for the subject.
- Knows the content well and has the appropriate level of clinical expertise.
- Uses the skills and procedures referred to in the lecture.
- Delivers a clear message including only what the course participants really need to know.
- Engages the course participants and uses appropriate body language.
- Keeps to time.
- Is available at break times to get to know course participants and answer questions.
- Liaises with faculty doing link discussions and practicals as well as other relevant lecturers, during the precourse.

Like most social skills, learning to teach involves using the talents you have, rather than trying to be what you are not. The skills and personality traits required by different teaching methods make conflicting demands. The extrovert lecturer who commands the attention of the course participants by occasional showmanship may have difficulty finding the sensitivity and responsiveness required to facilitate a discussion.

## 2 Before the course

## 2.1 Preparation

The eight recommended sequence of steps you should take after receiving an invitation to deliver a lecture:

1. Identify your message.
2. Set learning outcomes.
3. Develop the conclusion.
4. Build the main body.
5. Establish a catchy introduction.
6. Produce visual aids.
7. Edit content and number of slides.
8. Rehearse, rehearse, rehearse.

These steps are relevant whether you are a novice or experienced lecturer.

**Step 1: Identify your message**
What do you want course participants to do, be, feel, or know when they leave your lecture? If you answer this question in one sentence, make sure it is visible whenever you are working on the lecture and you will find it helps you to stay focused on the major issues.

**Step 2: Set learning outcomes**
Outcomes should be based on the major issues to be addressed. Are your course participants beginners, do they have some experience, or are they experts? Tailor the lecture content to the level of competence of the participants. If there is a related practical you should refer to it, but not in detail. The lecture should not be a vehicle for you to show off your expertise. What the course participants really need is to understand the overall message and put it to use.

### Step 3: Develop the conclusion

The conclusion is the last part of your lecture to be heard and the part the course participants are most likely to remember. Many successful lawyers exploit this. They write their final argument first, and then line up the evidence that best supports the facts they must prove to the jury.

Hovland et al [6] demonstrated that learners are more likely to accept a conclusion if the lecturer states it at the end of an argument. If the same evidence is presented with the conclusion left unstated, learners were unable to draw an inference from the lecture.

The conclusion should take about 5–10% of the overall presentation time (equivalent to 1–2 concluding slides). You can use it as the opportunity to summarize the 3–5 salient points. It is important to signal that you are nearing the end of your lecture. As soon as course participants hear "In conclusion…" or "Finally, let me repeat my main points…" they will listen more carefully. New issues should not be introduced at this point. If you are short of time never cut the conclusion; shorten the body of the lecture.

### Step 4: Build the main body

Russell et al [7] have shown that students learn more when information density is not too high. Miller [8] says that the average number of items of knowledge that a person can hold in their short-term memory is $7 \pm 2$. Once you have decided what you want to cover, it is tempting to squeeze too much into the session. If the content does not contribute to your main message, leave it out. Use the minimum number of facts, views, and opinions to convey it.

■ ⅲ    **Information overload is different from repeating the message. You should exclude details which will be delivered in a following practical exercise video.**

When dealing with data and figures: pick the first, largest, newest, latest, or smallest. If participants need more information, provide it in a handout afterwards. It is your job to take course participants behind the numbers and explain what they mean. Stick to the KISS principle (keep it short and simple). Use short words and short sentences. If participants have to struggle to understand any words or concepts, they are likely to give up **(Fig 6-1, Fig 6-2)**.

Use case illustrations which are common and relevant. It is worth collecting good slides of standard cases, which can be notoriously difficult to locate when you need them. Rare cases should be kept for experts or to illustrate a particular point. All cases should be made anonymous. Course participants appreciate and learn from a lecturer's openness about failures as well as successes.

Nelson [9] found that—compared to hypothetical examples—personal examples improved learners' attitudes toward the lecturer, increased their confidence, and increased their recall of the lecture material.

Throughout your lecture you should include "pep-me-ups". These can be anecdotes, interesting visuals, or bits of humor.

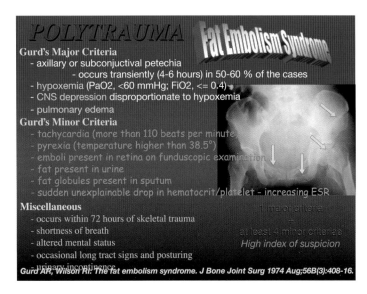

Fig 6-1    Example of a busy slide with inappropriate graphics crammed together.

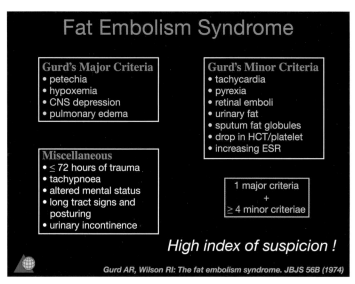

Fig 6-2    Example of a neat slide handling a lot of information.

## Step 5: Establish a catchy introduction

Your introduction is not the time to bore everyone with details of your curriculum vitae. You don't need to show irrelevant slides of your hospital or to thank anyone for asking you to lecture. Start straightaway with your opening sentence, not a tired old beginning like "Today, I'm going to talk about…".

This is your best chance to grab the course participants' attention. Within the first 2–4 minutes they will make up their mind about whether to listen to you. So, it is important to start with something memorable or attention grabbing: a short and interesting quote or an amazing slide **(Fig 6-3)**. During the rest of the introduction, it is important to identify what will be covered, how it links with the rest of the course and why it will be of interest.

## Step 6: Produce visual aids

Visual aids should be just that: visible and aids to your lecture. How many times have you heard a speaker using precious time to apologize for the clarity of a graphic? If the x-ray isn't clear don't show it, look for one in a textbook or download one from an Internet source.

Types of visual aids:

- Clinical photographs.
- X-rays.
- Line graphics.
- Bone models.
- Computer graphics.
- Video clips.
- Computer animations.

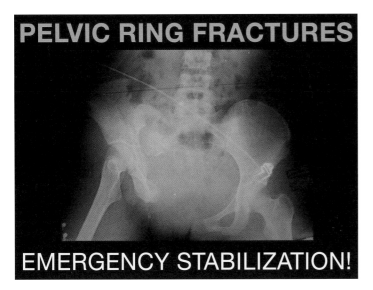
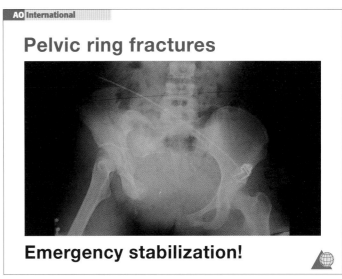

Fig 6-3    A catchy title slide which is self-explanatory—two different designs.

With the advent of complex computer programs, some untrained lecturers get carried away with the presentation of their slides or overhead transparencies. Sadly, course participants often leave such lectures impressed by the visual aids, but with no change in their understanding or opinion, and hence no learning. On the other hand, the digital revolution of the last decade has made quality clinical photography **(Table 6-1)** accessible to everyone [10].

The following principles should help you:

- One basic point per visual.
- Present figures as diagrams or graphs.
- Familiarize yourself with any equipment.
- Rehearse well with visual aids.
- No more than 15 slides for a 20-minute lecture.
- Show visual aids only when you are talking about them.
- Avoid using flowers, sunsets, or your children's photos to fill space.

| Scanning and photographing pictures and x-rays | |
|---|---|
| ■ Use digital cameras at high (XGA or 1024 × 768 pixels) or full (2048 × 1536 pixels) resolution; you can reduce them to 72 dpi later. | ■ Taking shots off an x-ray viewer may appear sharp on small 2-inch camera screens, yet result in shake blur when viewed on a larger (14-inch) computer screen; use elbow or tripod support. Beware reflections on newer glossy digital film. |
| ■ Output onto a computer or LCD projected screen is maximum 150 dpi; saving digital pictures at 300 dpi is useful if you are considering a future publication (print). | ■ Taking shots off a TV (fluoroscope) screen may result in a dark band across due to the 50-Hz flicker; set camera on Shutter-priority with speed at 1/15 to avoid this, but shake blur may occur at this speed; alternatively, photograph the printout. |
| ■ Use grayscale mode for x-rays and black-and-white graphics to save file size; also takes out blue-green tint from x-ray boxes. | ■ For best exposure of x-rays, center the focusing circle on the bony metaphysis or cancellous bone before recomposing. |
| ■ Scanning and photographing from glossy book pages may result in interference, Fresnel rings, or flare from overhead lighting (photocopy onto matt paper first); sometimes can be edited in Photoshop (Filter:Noise:Dust&scratches). | ■ When taking clinical or operative pictures, align to the vertical or horizontal axis to help the viewer orientate. |

Table 6-1   Tips for dealing with pictures.

If the feedback for your lecture is good, do consider donating your set of slides to the course chairman so future lecturers and course participants can benefit and your hard work will not be used on just one occasion.

### Step 7: Edit content and number of slides
At this stage of the preparation you will probably have too much content. What can be cut? What does not contribute to the overall message? Consider again the course participants you will be lecturing to. Are all the examples and cases relevant to their practice? Remember, the lecture on the course is likely to take at least 25% longer than during rehearsal. What elements can be cut if you run short of time on the day?

Once your lecture has been prepared, put it aside and return to it later. You will spot mistakes, confusing areas, and think of new ways of presenting. Remember, the greater your expertise, the more you need to structure and rehearse.

### Step 8: Rehearse
Don't try to learn the script by heart. Memorizing will get in the way of your flow. You will find yourself searching your memory for words rather than concentrating on delivering your message effectively. Rehearsal should take place at the venue, with your visual aids and notes, in real time. There is sometimes a temptation to miss this step and to read your lecture through a few times. This is not enough. An alternative is rehearsing to yourself in a mirror to check eye contact and timing. Rehearsing with a spouse or colleague also helps. Effective preparation for your lecture more than makes up for any lack of expertise or experience. It will also calm your nerves.

## 2.2    Using technology effectively

### 2.2.1    PowerPoint

This is the most commonly used computer presentation program for lectures. It is easy to use and has powerful tools, but some lecturers try to use all of them, when few are really needed to be effective. You may refer to the manual or countless other publications on PowerPoint but this is some practical advice to start with.

Useful features in PowerPoint include:

- Standard color schemes and backgrounds.
- Customizable text, fonts, and sizes.
- Drawing tools and clip arts.
- Easy insertion of graphic files, charts and tables, and video clips.
- A wide variety of animation tools.
- Ability to insert single slides or a whole lecture from your library.
- Ability to save as PowerPoint Show (.pps) file.

### Color schemes and background

Two basic schemes stand out in a presentation. First a white background, similar to using an overhead projector, with black text and diagrams, but is less effective when color graphics such as clinical pictures are added. X-rays alone stand out well.

Dark backgrounds work best: usually black or dark blue. Text will stand out if it is yellow, orange, or white. Avoid green and red as they do not project well. Remember that 10% of the male audience may have red/green color blindness. Graduated backgrounds should also be avoided due to poor contrast with text.

### Text fonts and sizes

Text size should be 20–36 point for visibility. Titles can be as large as 60 point. Sans serif fonts, eg, Arial and Helvetica, which are easy to read, are best. Avoid using more than two font types per slide. You can make letters bold for extra clarity. Avoid fancy WordArt as it can take time to load.

Here are some rules for slide text:

- Restrict the number of words to six across and six lines down.
- Spell everything correctly (try using Tools:Spelling or F7).
- For lists, keep text inside a box; you can reposition them anywhere.
- Use indents and bullets only one level down.
- Start with an "action" word and avoid full sentences.
- Avoid punctuation marks, unless it is a quote.
- The alignment function will help you line up texts vertically and horizontally.

### Drawing tools and clip arts

AutoShapes are useful in providing all manner of lines, basic shapes, block arrows, and flowcharts. You can re-size, rotate, and edit them. Lines can be used as curves or freehand. Closing allows them to be filled in color. You can Edit Points to outline, say, a bone on an x-ray and is best done by viewing the slide at 200–400% zoom.

### Insertion of graphic files, charts, tables, and video clips

As you prepare your outline, the lecture can be improved with graphics. You can explain the complex shape of a subtalar joint by showing it rather than by describing it.

An acetabular fracture can be better described in a 3-D CT-scan reconstruction, especially when you can rotate it. Such techniques will depend on your computer skills and are not essential. A diagram from a book may be enough. Just ask yourself "Is it visible and does it aid?"

■ ▥ **Sources of medical graphics:**

▥ **AO Image Collection PFxM, AO Teaching Support Kit, or other AO publications.**
▥ **Standard textbooks (difficulty with scanning glossy pages).**
▥ **Other donated lectures (acknowledge the contributor).**
▥ **CD-ROMs, web sources (www.primalpictures.com).**

Graphic files can seldom be inserted as they are taken and need to be processed. A drawing program such as Adobe Photoshop can be used to improve the image. You can change contrast and brightness, sharpen or crop, resize and change resolution. X-rays should be changed to grayscale to minimize file sizes and to maximize contrast. Similarly, line drawings or simple graphics with few colors can be saved in Index color mode to save space. You can insert graphics into PowerPoint as JPEG or TIF/TIFF files. Picture contrast, brightness, and cropping can also be done in PowerPoint itself (Picture:Toolbar). Experiment with size, but for computer presentation, a resolution of 72 dots per inch (dpi) is adequate. You may however wish to save them to your library at 300 dpi or higher if you are using it for a publication.

■ ▥ **Presenting graphics:**

▥ **X-rays should take up a quarter of the screen to be viewed clearly.**
▥ **People scan from left to right, so position text to the left of graphics.**
▥ **When using annotations, you can group graphics with text (Draw:Group) so they appear together.**

Charts and tables presented in publications are rarely suitable for projection without simplification. You may want to reproduce them by making your own chart and table within PowerPoint or Microsoft Word. The most common mistake is to make them too cluttered by data. Remember that participants are seeing it for the first time and for a very short time. Be prepared to explain the chart or diagram.

Video clips can be effective in showing steps of surgery or a functional outcome. When you are taking a video from a digital camera, keep the clip short. Lighting is also important especially with skin color, so set the camera to the right illumination, for example, fluorescent or incandescent light. Before inserting them into a slide, edit them to less than 20 seconds and save them in the same folder as your lecture file. Then you will remember where you put them and will transfer with the file when you save them to a CD-ROM or a memory stick.

■ ▥    **Tips for including video clips:**

▨ **PowerPoint works best with AVI files.**
▨ **You can use commercially available programs to prepare .avi files.**
▨ **Orientate the frame horizontally for video; it cannot be rotated.**
▨ **Short clips are best, especially to show steps of an operation.**
▨ **Inserted clips need to be linked to a file; transferring the PowerPoint file changes the link; clicking on the movie will prompt you to re-link it by finding the attached file.**
▨ **Handling video codes may differ with operating systems; download both the file and the video clip to the host computer; don't run from a data CD-ROM.**

### Animation

Animation effects can be overused and mask your message. However, it can be effective when developing the flow of an idea. With transparencies, the carousel must be advanced to go to the next page. In PowerPoint, you can use animation to show related images or text without changing slides until the page fills up. "Telling the story" becomes easier. You also control the pace that participants receive information and hold their attention and anticipation.

Rules for animation include:

▪ Limit Effects of animation and slide transition to two or less.
▪ Wipe Right or Wipe Down works well for text animation.
▪ Wipe directions must follow where an arrow points.
▪ Dissolve and Strips Right-Down are useful for graphics and x-rays.
▪ Text lines can be used as cue pointers.
▪ Intersperse text animation with graphics by grouping text with graphics.
▪ Flowcharts work very well with animation by following the rules above.
▪ Use By Mouse Click for starting animation for better control.
▪ Use Play settings to animate movie clips.
▪ Slide transitions are done in the Slide Sorter view; No Transition is best.

■ ▥    **Be careful:**

▨ **Automatic animations can be timed, but may disrupt flow in real time.**
▨ **Avoid using sounds during animations; they are irritating.**
▨ **Avoid selecting Random Effects for animations and Random Transitions for changing slides; they are very distracting.**
▨ **Not rehearsing with animations is dangerous; animation order changes when you add or delete text or graphics, and when you UnGroup and ReGroup graphics in the Draw menu.**

### Inserting slides from files

This is a powerful option to select single, a group of, or every slide from an existing PowerPoint file. You can do this in the Slide or SlideSorter views. The inserted slides will adopt the background of your current lecture. You may also copy and paste slides from the donor's SlideSorter view.

You should be aware that:

- Text fonts and size in inserted slides may change and reposition themselves.
- Fonts from another computer may not be found in the one you are using.
- Special characters may also change or be substituted.
- Text, line, and fill colors need to be changed to conform to the existing presentation.
- Contents may not be suitable or are repeated in the new lecture.
- Sometimes it is easier to copy and paste selected text or graphics between opened files than to import whole slides.
- If you use someone else's slide, give them credit.

### Saving your presentation

By default, PowerPoint will save your lecture as presentation (.ppt file). Try saving it as PowerPoint Show (.pps file) and place it on the desktop. When you double-click on it, your full-screen SlideShow will open without going through PowerPoint start-up. In fact, you don't even need the PowerPoint program to be installed on the host computer.

### 2.2.2 Laser or mouse pointers

Pointers should be used judiciously to target points on graphics, x-rays, or charts and draw the attention of the participants. They should not be used to point at text like the bouncing "karaoke" ball. If you have a hand tremor try resting your hand on the lectern.

A mouse arrow pointer in PowerPoint is another way of showing the participants what you want them to look at. If you click the left button the slide will advance; if you click the right button, an options menu will pop up and often disrupt your flow. It will only be useful when you want to skip to a specific slide. It is simplest to advance slides using the down arrow or PgDn key on the keyboard and move the mouse arrow as a pointer.

### 2.2.3 Audience response systems

Engaging a larger audience to interact and/or vote on case study options can be done in a number of simple cost-effective ways, such as a show of hands, or holding up red or green cards distributed with precourse materials. If resources allow, however, an audience response system (ARS) using touch pads is an effective method for maximizing interaction in a large audience setting (see 1 AO education—introduction).

## 3    During the course

Many good lecturers have failed to live up to their own expectations on the day. The course participants were perhaps not as receptive as expected after lunch, but maybe the lecturer could have used simple techniques to achieve success. The following tips will help you to deliver in 20 minutes, what you may have spent weeks or months preparing.

### 3.1    Preparing the environment

By checking the venue before the lecture is scheduled, you can sort out almost any problem, from faulty equipment to construction work outside. Trust nobody but yourself to check any equipment you might need. Check and double-check it. Make a contingency plan in case it fails at the last minute.

Today, many use computer presentations. If you do, do you know how to connect the video cable to the VGA (video graphics array) port of a laptop? Do you know what keystrokes are needed to interface the computer with the LCD (liquid crystal displays)? It is essential that technical expertise is available on the course if you do not have it yourself, so seek out the technician.

Be careful if you have prepared a CD-ROM or memory stick for your lecture. Keep the lecture file in a named folder. You must check it before uploading. Always keep the original with you as backup. Video clips can be a particular problem.

Room lighting should be kept bright to maintain course participants' attention. If this proves difficult to view the screen, ask for technical support or consider removing light bulbs at the front of the room near the screen. It is worth checking the seating layout to see whether any changes will help participants see better.

### 3.2    Positioning yourself

If possible standing to your left of the screen makes it comfortable for course participants to read the slide and turn their eyes to you. It is important to stand up, allowing you to breathe more easily, to project your voice, and to maintain attention. It's all right to walk about the room, as long as your movements are purposeful. Control pointless wandering and rocking while speaking.

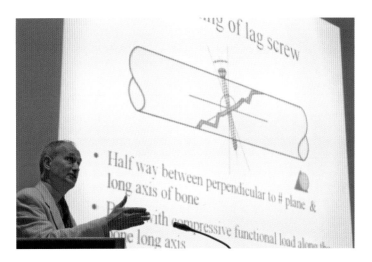

Fig 6-4    Communicate with your whole being.

### 3.3 Body language and eye contact

The best lecturers communicate with their whole being (**Fig 6-4**). They are animated and exciting to watch. However, many people are too inhibited to be able to use themselves deliberately as a visual aid. The role of body language in communication has increased in profile during the 1990s, although there are differing views about the significance of this nonverbal communication.

Albert Mehrabian, professor of psychology at the University of California, has calculated that only about 7% of understanding comes from what is actually said, 38% coming from the tone of voice, and 55% from nonverbal cues [11].

Certainly, if you are able to read other people's body language and use your own, you can establish rapport more quickly and effectively with others. Conversely, if you allow your body language to leak messages about some of your emotions, for example, disgust, fear, or irritation, such rapport becomes difficult.

Body posture is important, as it signals attention and respect to the group. In Western cultures this means leaning the upper body towards the group, showing an engaged body posture. By keeping your chin up, you will be able to maintain good eye contact and indicate confidence and interest. Coats et al [12] have shown that eye contact is important in establishing rapport with learners. Poor eye contact can give the impression of anxiety, incompetence, lack of sincerity, lack of credibility, and it prevents you from eliciting feedback from course participants.

However, in certain cultures, for example, Asian, locking eyes may cause the recipient to avert their gaze. Sweeping across the room, with short stops at individuals may be less intimidating. One cardinal rule is to avoid speaking without eye contact.

■ ▦ **Generating interactivity:**

**Buzz groups are groups of 2–6 participants who discuss issues or problems for short periods within a lecture. Such interactivity can have a significant impact on learning.**
**Several times after significant points were made in a lecture, Hollingsworth [13] instructed learners to discuss for 2 minutes what they thought was most important. Compared with a control group, these learners listened more attentively and—although their advantage was insignificant on a delayed test—they scored significantly higher on an immediate posttest.**

### 3.4 Voice

It is through voice and language that you transmit your message, so speak more slowly than usual to the back of the room. Practice speaking into a tape recorder and listen to yourself. Sazar et al [14] discovered that profanities had a negative effect on the acquisition of content and cooperation during the lecture.

■ ▦    **Beware of:**

▦    **Speech slurry—"ums" and "ers" get in the way; eventually people will become so distracted, they start to count these useless fillers.**

▦    **Filler words are a problem—three favorite fillers are "generally speaking", "actual", and "basically"; you may have other words you slip in when you're not thinking.**

▦    **Any bad language, expletive or discriminatory remarks—if in doubt, leave it out.**

▦    **Repetition, which is the mother of retention— make sure any repetition covers important points.**

▦    **Dropping your voice at the end of a sentence—this becomes difficult to listen to, and content is lost.**

▦    **Slurred or mumbled words, which will eventually irritate, as course participants will have to strain to understand you.**

▦    **Failure to pause long enough between ideas.**

Listeners need time to reflect on what they have heard. This is particularly important if you are addressing an audience whose first language is not the one you are speaking. Sometimes, it may even be necessary to leave out difficult concepts for discussions. Periods of silence or prolonged pauses are useful to regain course participants' attention. It also gives them time to absorb an important point. Such silences can be as long as 5–6 seconds, without feeling uncomfortable. Morgan et al [15] confirm that pauses at the end of sentences promote the "thinking time" so crucial for understanding.

Pace of presentation—ie, how quickly or slowly you speak—makes a difference as well. Geller et al [16] manipulated lecture speeds and used an ARS to provide feedback about when a lecturer was going too fast or too slow. Learners hardly ever indicated that the lecturer was going too slow.

### 3.5    Notes

If notes help you feel more confident and stay focused, prepare them carefully and use them with skill.

■ ▦    **Some tips on preparing notes:**

▦    **Using index cards makes it easier to rearrange.**

▦    **Only put in keywords to prompt you.**

▦    **Write large text so you can see in dim lighting.**

▦    **Punch a hole in a corner and tie with a string or clip in case you drop the pile.**

▦    **Keywords on the slide itself can also substitute for cards.**

Notes can be particularly helpful if the language of your lecture is not your first. However, when you read from a script, it is always frustrating for course participants. We can read at approximately 500 words a minute, whereas we can only speak at around 100. By reading from a script you lose spontaneity and interaction. Your head will be bowed, making eye contact impossible, voice projection difficult, and it is easy to lose your place in the notes. Meanwhile the course participants have drifted off. Coats et al [12] have shown that lecturers are more effective when they speak around a few points than when a lecture is read.

### 3.6 Using humor

People like laughing. People tend to like people who make them laugh, and if they like you, they will usually listen more carefully to what you say. However, a positive and enthusiastic approach is much more valuable than being able to tell jokes confidently. Amusing real life stories can relieve tension and help people learn. Avoid joking about sex, race, language, or religion. One insensitive or irrelevant remark can lose the course participants. To open the lecture with a joke takes skill and is a risk. Unless you are confident that you will be able to handle the situation if it falls flat, don't take that risk.

■ ▦ **Would you feel comfortable telling the joke or story**...
> ...**to your mother or grandmother?**
> ...**to a religious leader?**
> ...**if it were to be broadcast to the whole country?**
> ...**to everyone in the coffee room at lunchtime?**

Bryant et al [17] reported that humor enhanced student's approval of male lecturers but had the opposite effect with female lecturers, except when the humor was at someone else's expense. Humor appears to make no difference to recall immediately after the lecture, but if it is relevant and related to the point being explained, it improves recall later [18].

### 3.7 Managing special circumstances
### 3.7.1 Laptop/desktop does not work

If your own laptop refuses to cooperate, it may be:

- The power adapter is not plugged in and you have run out of battery.
- You ejected a CD-ROM, memory stick, or PC card during a read process.
- If your screen went blank, try pressing Fn and F7 (or F5) a few times to change output to the screen or projector (wait a while for the effect).

Whatever the difficulty, do not force the participants to share your frustrations. Ask them to work with the person next to them on a problem or exercise related to your lecture. Perhaps they could pose questions for themselves and then seek answers from the lecture. Otherwise, they could discuss their own clinical experience of your topic. The moderator could also help by asking questions.

King [19] reported that learners posing questions to themselves at the beginning of a lecture learned and remembered more in the long run than learners who took their own notes or who were given handouts.

Meanwhile you can attempt to rectify the technical problem. Have a contingency plan to cope if your visual aids are irretrievable and the technical staff have to take over: another good reason to have prepared notes. Having a standby computer with your lecture loaded is best. Transparencies for overhead projection can also be helpful but seldom necessary.

To minimize this risk, you should:

- Bring your power adapter even if your battery is fully charged.
- Power-up your computer a few minutes before you are to speak.
- Load and check the lecture file—and then leave everything on.
- Close all unnecessary screen windows and programs.
- Have a backup computer, CD-ROM, diskette, or memory stick.

### 3.7.2    Projector does not work

The problem could be with the projector or your computer. Compatibility and sync problems are rarer nowadays but you should know what to do, especially if you are using your own computer. Such preparation should take place long before the lecture is due to start, possibly first thing in the morning, during breaks, or at lunch.

Some projectors may go on "standby" mode and will need a minute to warm up when you want to use them. Look for the blinking green light on top of the projector. Warn your technician to turn on the machine if you don't have the controls. If you see the projector brand name on the screen after you connect, press Fn and F7 (or F5) key three times to switch display screens. You should then be able to see your own laptop screen. If not, press the "source" button on the projector to "refresh" from "video" back to "computer".

### 3.7.3    Different cultures and languages

AO is a worldwide organization with all the benefits of working with clinicians from different cultures and countries. However, it can be difficult to be sensitive to the differences between us.

- Always check with the local organizer about the proficiency of the participants in the language in which you will be speaking, usually English. Be aware that some cultures are unwilling to confess to ignorance. Local organizers will always estimate the ability of the audience to understand English.
- Check for any possible differences in clinical practice, eg, availability of C-arm.
- Try to find out more about the host country before you leave or upon arrival.
- Reduce your speaking speed, so your lecture will take longer, and thus require fewer slides; clever local course chairmen give a longer time slot for each lecture.
- Strictly avoid colloquialisms, culture-specific stories, and jokes which will not make sense to the participants.
- More time will be required to understand messages from slides; consider providing handouts of the outline before your lecture.
- Illustrations in the form of graphics, animations, clinical photographs, or x-rays will reinforce understanding.
- If a translator is provided take time out before your presentation to discuss it with him. Translators may be unfamiliar with some medical terms, and the best translators will always ask you to go through your presentation in advance with them, so that difficulties can be avoided.

- Be aware that there are possible cultural taboos, eg, showing of parts of the anatomy in a clinical slide, misinterpretation of a jocular slide showing religious or political content; if in doubt, leave it out.
- You may be showing techniques and technology unfamiliar to the course participants; balance the way you do things and propose an alternative where appropriate.
- Always be available during the whole course as course participants may be unwilling to ask questions openly during the lecture.
- Beware of targeting questions to senior members of the course who may "lose face" in front of their subordinates if they are unable to answer correctly.
- Practicals and discussions are key activities to assess the practice of course participants who may have developed novel ways for managing certain conditions despite lack of resources.
- Show humility and give credit to the local organizers or senior (often older) course participants who may be part of a hierarchical society.
- As foreign faculty you are often held in high esteem and have the responsibility for influencing clinical practice.

### 3.7.4 Handling hostility

Many lecturers dread the prospect of a "difficult course participant". In reality, of course, the vast majority of learners want you to succeed as they want to learn from you. However, there may be times when people disagree with our message. Whenever people disagree, it is difficult to see the other person's point of view. As faculty, it is essential that you try to understand and to minimize potential damage.

Carl Rogers [20] describes "unconditional positive regard". He argued that this quality, the ability to accept another person without judgment, is essential for learning to proceed and change to occur. So, in addition to teaching skills, faculty should not forget to bring sensitivity and respect to the courses and their lectures.

When dealing with difficult course participants, your goals are to:

- Get the difficult person on board.
- Minimize negative impact on any other course participants.
- Minimize time overrun.

■ ▦ **Tips:**

- ▦ **Always face a difficult situation straight away.**
- ▦ **Never embarrass anyone in front of the group.**
- ▦ **Never show you are angry during a lecture.**
- ▦ **Concentrate on the audience not yourself.**
- ▦ **Start your clarification from a point you both agree with.**

Very occasionally you may be faced with a hostile course participant. Sometimes they appear uninformed and apathetic. For these individuals it is essential to grab their attention early on. Information needs to be carefully explained, given a little at a time, repeated with variations and with plenty of examples. Stress your own expertise and use lots of successful role models and examples.

Even though there may be faculty and course participants who are experts in your field, they are NOT an expert in what you are going to talk about. We frequently attend lectures in our area of expertise, but seldom come away from one having learned nothing at all. We always learn a new tip or an interesting case. We also discover new ways of explaining difficult areas, which we can later use with other participants.

### 3.7.5   Cutting the lecture short
Preferably you will finish before the end of your time slot, rather than running overtime when course participants will start to fidget and wonder whether their whole day will then run late. No matter how tempting, it is arrogant to assume that what you have to say takes priority. If you run late then tight schedules fall into disarray. Anyway, you should remember that the average student's attention span is between 10 and 20 minutes [21].

Plan your timings on the premise that your lecture on the day will take 25–50 % longer than your rehearsal to allow time for entertaining questions from course participants and for the inevitable slippage in large groups [22]. Be prepared to make cuts if your time is short, but do not cut the introduction or conclusion. An easy way to accomplish this is to color code your lecture into three sections:

- Must know.
- Should know.
- Could know.

### 3.7.6   Managing interactive debates
Interactive debates are becoming increasingly common. Many topics work well as a debate, for example, intramedullary nailing versus minimally invasive plating for diaphyseal fractures. You should liaise early with the course chairman, moderator, and any other faculty involved. Preparing your arguments in advance is important. Sometimes it is tempting to make outrageous contributions with the aim of influencing course participants to support your view, or to make them laugh. On the other hand, with poor preparation the debater's arguments may be weak or unconvincing. Participants are looking for the contest in arguments. However, the educational strength of this method lies with a balanced view and transparent thought processes which help course participants to develop their own decision-making skills and hone their judgment.

### 3.7.7   Role as a session moderator
You may be invited to be a session moderator in addition to delivering a lecture. In the past, a moderator's job was to introduce the speaker and to keep the session to time. Good moderators have used their own initiatives to liven up the session by posing questions and encouraging audience response, but this is often erratic and inconsistent.

The role of a session moderator can help enhance the learning process. They are usually experienced senior faculty who have a sound overview of the area being covered. They should:

- Coordinate with speakers long beforehand to ensure no duplication of content.
- Work with speakers to present appropriate case studies.
- Prepare ARS case studies to involve audience participation and engage the speakers.
- Be decisive in cutting short lectures which exceed the time limit.
- Be able to sum up the key learning points of that session.

## 4     After the course

Most AO courses adopt a form of course evaluation. Course participants may be asked to assess your lecture according to set criteria. Such criteria include organization, evidence base, presentation style, etc. Such evaluation will probably tell you little that you did not know already, but it is useful for chairmen in assessing the value of including a particular lecture in a future course.

Self-evaluation is probably the most useful way to improve your own performance. Shortly after your presentation, write down the three most successful elements of the lecture. Next, write down the three things you would change, if you were asked to repeat the lecture.

■ ▥     **Feedback is the fuel that drives improved performance.**

## 5     Conclusion

The essence of a good lecture is not so much in the content but in the preparation and attention to detail. You must know what it takes to deliver a good lecture, to provide just the right amount and level of content, to engage course participants, to summarize the key points, and to elicit feedback to improve the next lecture.

Remember these key points when you prepare your lecture:

- What is the message participants need to remember from you?
- Effective lectures need meticulous preparation.
- Focus on introduction and conclusion.
- No more than five major points.
- Course participants cannot learn everything in a lecture.
- Brutal editing improves flow and ensures good time keeping.
- Do not allow visual aids to drive your lecture.

## 6     Anecdote

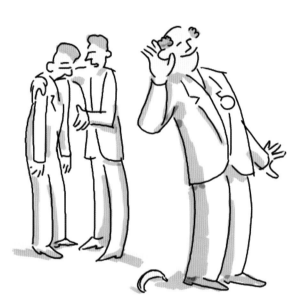

*As Jacob assumed a more senior role on course faculty, his anxiety increased before and during his lectures. Despite trying relaxation techniques, avoiding caffeine, eating bananas, and even resorting to beta-blockers, he found the symptoms he experienced more and more difficult to quell. His hands shook, his voice was not his own, his mouth dried, and his pulse raced.*

*Just before, what he had decided was to be, his final course, he heard a conversation between two more junior faculty members.*

*"I get really nervous before these courses."*
*"Why?"*
*"In case something goes wrong."*
*"What like?"*
*"Well...I don't know...my mind goes blank or someone asks me a question I don't know the answer to..."*
*"Why would that be so terrible?"*
*"Well...I'd look really stupid."*
*"Only if you behaved stupidly."*
*"It's not that simple."*
*"Oh, I think it is. Participants are here to learn something from you. They've not come to see how clever, knowledgeable, and skilled you are. In fact they're not that interested in you. They need something which will help them care for patients better."*

*Overhearing that conversation helped Jacob refocus on what mattered. His job was to prepare as well as he could, so that learners would learn what they needed to. By shifting the focus from himself onto course participants, not only did he do a better job, but his anxiety diminished to easily controllable levels.*

*Lisa Hadfield-Law*

## 7    Bibliography

1. **Smeltzer L, Watson K** (1983) *Improving listening skills used in business*: American Business Communication Association.

2. **Cotton J** (1995) *The Theory of Learning Strategies: an introduction*. Philadelphia: Kogan Page.

3. **Davis D, Evans M, Jadad A, et al** (2003) The case for knowledge translation: shortening the journey from evidence to effect. *BMJ*; 327(7405):33–35.

4. **Grimshaw JM, Shirran L, Thomas R, et al** (2001) Changing provider behavior: an overview of systematic reviews of interventions. *Med Care*; 39(8):II2–45.

5. **Bligh DA** (2000) *What's the use of lectures?* San Francisco: Jossey-Bass Publishers.

6. **Hovland CI, Mandell W** (1952) An experimental comparison of conclusion-drawing by the communicator and by the audience. *J Abnorm Psychol*; 47(3):581–588.

7. **Russell IJ, Hendricson WD, Herbert RJ** (1984) Effects of lecture information density on medical student achievement. *J Med Educ*; 59(11):881–889.

8. **Miller G** (1967) *The Psychology of Communication*. New York: Penguin.

9. **Nelson G** (1992) The relationship between the use of personal, cultural examples in international teaching assistants' lectures and uncertainty reduction, student attitude, student recall, and ethnocentrism. *International Journal of Intercultural Relations*; 16(1):33–52.

10. **Niamtu J** (2004) Image is everything: pearls and pitfalls of digital photography and PowerPoint presentations for the cosmetic surgeon. *Dermatol Surg*; 30(1):81–91.

11. **Mehrabian A** (1972) *Non-Verbal Communication*. Chicago: Aldine Atherton.

12. **Coats W, Smidchens U** (1966) Audience recall as a function on speaker dynamism. *Journal of Educational Psychology*; 57(4):189–191.

13. **Hollingsworth P** (1995) Enhancing listening retention: the two-minute discussion. *College Student Journal*; 29(1):116–117.

14. **Sazar L, Kassinove H** (1991) Effects of counselor's profanity and subject's religiosity on content acquisition of a counseling lecture and behavioural compliance. *Psychological Reports*; 69(3):1059–1070.

15. **Morgan S, Puglisi J** (1982) Enhancing memory for lecture sentences: a depth perspective. *Pathological Reports*; 51(2):675–678.

16. **Geller E, Chaffee J, Farris J** (1975) Research in modifying lecturer behaviour with continuous student feedback. *Educational Technology*; 15(12):31–35.

17. **Bryant J, Comiski P, Cime J, et al** (1980) The relationship between college teachers use of humor in the class room and student's evaluation of their teachers. *Journal of Educational Psychology*; 72(4):511–519.

18. **Javidi M, Long L** (1989) Teacher's use of humor, self disclosure, and narrative activity as a function of experience. *Communication Research Reports*; 6(1):47–52.

19. **King A** (1992) Facilitating elaborative learning through guided student generated questioning. *Educational Psychologist*; 27(1):111–126.

20. **Rogers CR** (1951) *Client-Centered Counseling*. Boston: Houghton-Mifflin.

21. **Penner JG** (1984) *Why Many College Teachers Cannot Lecture*. Springfield: Thomas.

22. **Christensen N** (1988) "Nuts and Bolts of Running a Lecture Course." *Deneff AL, Goodwin CD, McCrate ES (eds). The Academic Handbook*. Durham: Duke University Press.

# 7    How to run an operating room personnel (ORP) course

## 1    Introduction

Training operating room personnel (ORP) has been an integral part of AO's educational strategy since its inception in 1961. AO pioneers recognized that the role of the nurse would be crucial in achieving the best patient outcomes, underpinned by AO principles and philosophy. At early courses, nurse participants assisted surgeons during their osteosynthesis practicals, which mirrored practice in the operating theater. However, course organizers soon recognized that the educational needs of nurses would be much better met if they themselves did the practicals (practical exercises). Being able to use the tools would help them assemble and understand the sequence of instrumentation. Lectures were also delivered by surgeons, but not ORP, in order to provide the theoretical background to the fixations of fractures used in the practicals.

Today, AO courses for ORP are designed to increase their competence in the pre-, peri-, and postoperative phase of fracture management. Courses help them assume their unique role in caring for these patients. ORP must be able to identify instrumentation, assemble and maintain it, know how it works, and understand the sequence in which it is used. The skills required to effectively teach an ORP course are very similar to those required on a surgeon's course. Faculty members, therefore, will need to read previous chapters covering relevant responsibilities on ORP courses. The purpose of this chapter is to explore special aspects of teaching ORP, on a worldwide basis.

## 1.1    Outcomes

By the end of this chapter the reader will be able to:

- **Define the roles of ORP.**
- **Identify how ORP learning needs differ from surgeons.**
- **Evaluate the specific needs of ORP on AO courses including lectures, practicals, and discussions.**
- **Consider the effects of diversity, including culture and gender, on learning.**
- **Plan their contribution as ORP faculty and potential mentor/mentee.**
- **Explore how coaching can support learning on ORP courses.**
- **Discuss the role of reflection on courses.**

## 2 What is the role of the ORP?

Since the late 1980s several trends have emerged to change the traditional face of nursing, including a change in the public's perception, a rise in the number of men in nursing and women in medicine, the constant problem of nursing shortages and new roles in health care which promote specialist and advanced practice.

ORP function at a variety of levels depending on where they work, their speciality, their years of experience, and work environment. In the United States, the roles of registered nurse first assistants (RNFA), the perioperative nurse practitioner, and the perioperative clinical nurse specialist (CNS) have developed to provide care to surgical patients. The role of RNFAs, like the role of the surgical practitioner in the UK, is constantly evolving, and this evolution continually changes day-to-day practice of the specialist ORP in the workplace.

■ ▥ **Faculty should, however, remember that not all ORP are registered nurses and they tend to practice differently throughout the world.**

### 2.1 Diversity

In many countries of the world ORP's function is to assist the surgeon. In a few countries the role has been expanded or even changed, resulting in advanced practice roles. As faculty it is important to find out as much as you can about the culture in which surgery is practiced. Culture within this context can be defined as an individual's character and belief system, as influenced by race, ethnicity, religion, gender, social status, and environment [1]. It is inappropriate and insensitive to assume that those you will be teaching work in the same way as you, or have access to similar resources. Even when teaching in your own area, with globalization, countries are experiencing diversity in the composition of their population, and hence, their workforce.

■ ▥ **When teaching in regional ORP courses, make sure to understand the culture and the current and future roles of the ORP learners.**

Although the importance of understanding diversity when caring for patients has been debated at length, there has been little discussion about how to incorporate cultural, age, and gender diversity into education. As a start, faculty should examine their own prejudice and bias, although this will not be easy, as most people are fairly blind to their bias or ethnocentric perspectives [2]. It may help to identify a peer coach from a different cultural group, gender, professional background, or age bracket. They can provide feedback on your teaching performance and materials, and can help you identify omissions or uncover stereotypes. By selecting a peer coach or mentor from a different group, but teaching on the same course, a more cohesive faculty will be created.

Prejudice and bias can be serious obstacles to learning. Stereotyping occurs when there is an untruth or an oversimplification of traits and behaviors common to an entire group of people. Stereotypes can refer to a number of variables, such as physical appearance, intellectual attributes, personality characteristics, career roles, domestic roles, social placement, gender, or ethnicity.

■ ⫶     **One common linguistic bias concerns the use of feminine pronouns for nurses and male pronouns for surgeons.**

Many find such labeling inappropriate, or even insulting. When a course participant is offended, they are likely to share their negative feelings with others, which will hinder their ability to concentrate on the content and learn from it. The protagonists may also find themselves isolated and unable to engage with learners.

To broaden cultural perspectives, ORP and surgeon faculty should take as many opportunities as possible to spend unstructured parts of the course with other cultural groups. It is tempting to mix with friends and close colleagues during coffee breaks and at the course dinner. However, these opportunities can help you understand the norms and values of others, as well as the contexts in which they practice.

ORP participants, and indeed some of the surgeon participants, may not have been in a formal learning environment for some time. Rogers [3] points out that some adults re-entering education after time away expect to be treated like children and are therefore inclined to be passive. He is, however, of the opinion that eventually they will rebel against such passive learning and even suggests provoking such a situation in order to secure greater participation in the education process. As faculty, you may need to anticipate such challenges and plan how you might handle them beforehand. It would be unrealistic to expect this type of learner to immediately engage in a balanced and fruitful group discussion. You will need to consider how to build trust and help partici-

pants feel comfortable in the early part of the course, so that learners feel safe to fully participate and can then respond positively to gentle provocation and challenge.

■ ⫶     **Creating a culturally sensitive learning environment requires more than just support for course participants; it also requires support for the faculty. Thus, course chairmen and organizers share this responsibility through their leadership, the structure of programs, and social activities [4].**

### 3    How do ORP courses differ from surgeons' courses?

One common mistake made by first time faculty is to teach on an ORP course as though it were a surgeon's course. Although there are a number of similarities, it is important to return to the planning stage of any session with which you are involved and consider both content and delivery.

■ ▥    **Think carefully about the learners on the course. What is the clinical context in which they work?**

### 3.1    Practicals

ORP around the world are primarily concerned with how their role contributes to effective patient care. They need to be familiar with the instrumentation required to achieve fracture fixation: the techniques of instrument assembly and the sequence in which they are used. Because the instrumentation is so important to ORP course participants, they need more time to handle the instruments before the practical can begin. The surgeons' teaching videos provide minimal coverage of the instrumentation, and practical directors may find it helpful to run through the instruments, on the CCTV (closed-circuit television), in the order in which they are used, before the practical starts. The practical should be directed by an ORP faculty member with a surgical faculty member. This combination achieves the appropriate balance between the skills involved in instrument handling and assembly and the skills involved in fracture fixation. Successful partnerships clearly agree upon their roles well in advance. When a practical session does not work well, it is usually due to lack of preparation.

■ ▥    **The best team to present a practical in an ORP course consists of an ORP and a surgeon who have agreed on their respective roles before the practical begins.**

The table instructor's role is crucial during these sessions, as they are in a good position to make sure participants are able to handle the instruments appropriately **(Fig 7-1)**. It is particularly important that they use the small groups at the tables as a vehicle, and make sure all members of the group are engaged in the activities. Table instructors should be aware that, although ORP may have limited experience in using instruments, they have a great deal of experience in assembling them. The focus should, therefore, be placed on how the instruments are used during surgery.

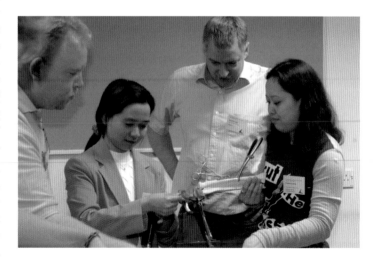

Fig 7-1    Good teamwork makes the practical learning experience successful.

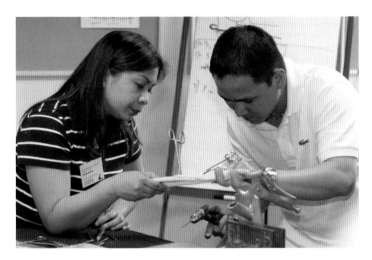

Fig 7-2    Enough time for practicals is needed to successfully accomplish the exercises.

ORP must have enough time to complete practical exercises than surgeons, as they are less familiar with the skills needed to use the instrumentation **(Fig 7-2)**. ORP and surgeons become demoralized when they cannot complete fracture fixation during a session; so sufficient allocation of time is crucial. It is a common observation that ORP participants tend to follow instructions more carefully than their surgical colleagues, often resulting in greater accuracy with regard to their final fixation.

### 3.2    The effect of gender on psychomotor performance

The effect of gender on psychomotor performance is still controversial, however, objective evidence on the matter is limited. Grantcharov et al [5] showed no difference in performance between male and female surgical trainees, based on performance in virtual reality laparoscopy. However, this is not consistent with the findings reported in previous studies of open surgery [6]. In this study, female surgical trainees showed superior academic achievement compared with their male counterparts. However, in comparison to male controls, female trainees received consistently lower surgical-skills ratings, particularly on items measuring confidence and task organization. When considered in the context of AO courses, and particularly ORP courses, these findings suggest differences between genders, which may need to be taken into consideration by faculty when considering timing and supervision during courses.

### 3.3    Discussion groups

ORP work and learn in small groups, so conventional wisdom might suggest that they would find discussion groups useful on courses. However, this does not seem to be the case around the world, as many course participants find the small group environment uncomfortable. There may also be language barriers. To get the most from these sessions, it is important to assemble the discussion group members as early in the course as possible. An ideal opportunity is to gather each group together, either at course registration or during the first coffee break. By meeting together in a social situation, many of the barriers can start being dismantled **(Fig 7-3)**.

Participants need to be clear about what is expected of them during discussions. They also need to know what contribution can be expected from participating faculty. Surgeon and ORP faculty commonly moderate group discussion sessions together, which can work well. However, there is a danger that the surgeon will dominate the discussion group, forcing others to take a

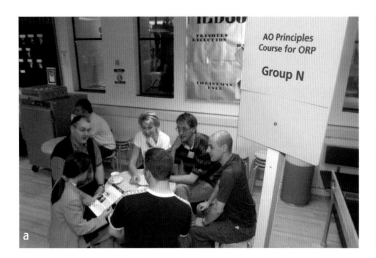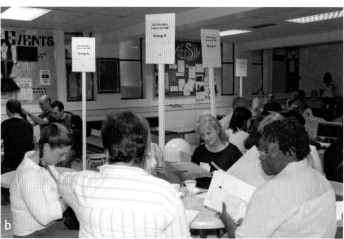

Fig 7-3a–b    Meeting of the discussion groups at a very early stage of the course—after registration or during first coffee break. They get to know each other and become familiar with the roles they will have to adopt during the course.

passive role. In some cultures, ORP, or those considered more junior, are unwilling to express their own opinion when a surgeon is present. These cultural issues must be considered when planning and leading a discussion in many parts of the world.

■ ▥    **If a surgeon within a discussion group takes on a dominant role, it will interfere with effective learning.**

If surgical faculty is to be included in an ORP group, clarity of roles is, again, crucial before the discussion starts. ORP faculty often has the skills to facilitate discussion, and surgeons can be useful as an expert resource rather than the facilitator. Remember that ORP find these sessions useful for discussion of their own experiences in caring for patients with fractures.

### 3.4    Lectures

The content of lectures given on ORP courses should differ from those on surgeons' courses. The focus should be on preparing the patient for surgery and the instrumentation. Although ORP do need to understand the theoretical background for any surgical intervention, they do not need detailed anatomy, physiology, and biomechanics. Faculty members sometimes try to use a lecture prepared for a surgeon's course on an ORP course or, even worse, they invite ORP to sit in on a session at the surgeons' course. Although shared learning is considered to be an effective way of improving teamwork, ORP should not be deprived of the opportunity to focus on issues pertaining to their own role, including patient positioning, infection control, and the care and maintenance of equipment. Some ORP are now involved in decision making at preoperative planning meetings, which may mean some consideration of surgical aspects is important for them.

- ∎ ▥    **Shared learning is considered to be an effective way of improving teamwork between surgeons and ORP—but, the focus of the ORP's teaching should be on what they need to know in order to do a better job.**

ORP prefer lectures covering ORP issues to be given by ORP and surgical content to be given by surgeons, such as the indications for bridge plating. However, ORP faculty members are often less confident in their presentation skills. Surgeons have usually been expected to give presentations throughout their training and tend to feel more confident in this situation, whereas ORP are less likely to have addressed large groups of people. ORP may require help to access appropriate training and support. Peer coaching between ORP and surgeons (see 7 How to run an ORP course; 4.1 Coaching and mentoring on ORP courses) may also provide an excellent opportunity to improve skills and establish relationships.

## 4    Working with ORP faculty

Hitchcock et al [7] pointed out that in addition to training in teaching methods, faculty need opportunities to develop networks of colleagues, find appropriate mentors, and understand the fundamentals of faculty life. General educational research has shown these needs to be more acute for women and minority faculty [8]. It can be tempting to seek out fellow teachers from your own professional background during courses. However, in the interests of creating an integrated and effective faculty, it is important to resist such temptation. Mentoring programs can help.

Teaching on ORP courses may well involve fellow faculty and participants from around the world. Karle [9] identified a number of dissimilarities between regions and countries regarding the basic conditions for clinical education. These are explained by differences in teaching tradition, cultural and socioeconomic conditions, the health and disease spectrum of the region, and national organizations of health care delivery. However, he was astonished to find that, contrary to what would be expected from these variations in background and approaches, similarities most often prevail over the differences.

Despite these similarities, it is important to familiarize yourself with the values and experiences of different groups, and not just those from different countries. Given the gender stereotypes surrounding medicine, nursing, and other ORP [10, 11], the shift from traditional to modern views of health care professionals may be uncomfortable and radical to some.

### 4.1 Coaching and mentoring on ORP courses

Faculty teaching on courses for the first time can feel anxious and isolated. ORP tend to be more open than surgeons about their anxieties, and can, therefore, be easier to help and support. One successful initiative on ORP courses has been with peer coaching.

Peer coaching was introduced by Joyce and Showers [12]. They discovered that participation in peer coaching teams had a dramatic impact on the transfer and application of new learning. Teachers who received training in theory, combined with demonstration, practice, and participation in peer coaching study teams, showed an 80% transfer and application of new learning [13].

A peer review program with AO surgical faculty in the UK had mixed results. While faculty was happy to receive feedback from a medical educator, some were less willing to ask for and accept feedback from colleagues or juniors, who they considered to lack the appropriate expertise. Similar initiatives with ORP, though, proved more successful.

### 4.2 Assuming a mentorship role

By establishing a mentor program within courses, new faculty members have a point of contact and can access feedback. Mentoring is a skill in itself and requires some preparation. If course chairmen can appoint mentors, where required, a couple of weeks before the course, faculty can start to establish a relationship with their mentees before they even meet. By making contact, you can both decide what kind of support is required. Some will want help in preparation; others will only require feedback as they go along and advice on any problems.

Most will appreciate guidance on where to go and what to do. Decide early when, how often, and where you will meet during the course.

■ ▪ **When mentoring, it is important to understand the distinction between counseling and advising and, wherever possible, encourage your colleague to work out their own solutions with you acting only as a sounding board. Remember that you will be a role model and how you are seen to manage in situations on the course will affect the relationship you have with the mentee and how they assume the role of faculty member.**

Any feedback you give should be clear, honest, constructive, and designed to build confidence and ongoing commitment in your colleague. Feedback to the course chairman about your mentees' progress will help with planning, during and after the course. You might also want to consider using this relationship to access some feedback for yourself about your own teaching.

## 5    Breaking down hierarchical barriers

Sometimes ORP course faculty and participants complain that the steep hierarchical gradient encountered on courses interferes with effective learning. A paternalistic approach—where the teacher "tells" the learner what to know, be, do, or feel—forces the learner to be over-dependent. Knowles [14] argues that the point at which people take responsibility for their own growth and development is the point at which they become psychologically adult. It could be argued that "reaching adulthood" should be an essential prerequisite for safe surgical practice. So, how can faculty encourage participants to take responsibility for their learning, or at least share it? Moreover, how can this be achieved within a course lasting a few days, when barriers have built up over a long period of time? The answer is, of course, that they can't. However, all faculty members can make sure that they avoid any behaviors or comments that reinforce the traditional stereotypes of surgical omnipotence [15] and ORP subservience. They can also take every opportunity to flatten any type of hierarchy in evidence on the course. A good example concerns how faculty and participants address each other: consistency, whether using first names or not, is essential.

## 6    Development of ORP courses

An invaluable ingredient in any ORP educational event is the opportunity for cultural exchange among the participants, and between the participants and faculty. The exchange of information and the sharing of experiences will be of the utmost importance in order to prevent superfluous efforts in trying to reinvent the wheel and to spread good practice. It is therefore vital that course programs provide as many opportunities for interaction as possible.

To ensure a future for ORP training, new members of the faculty are essential. In the past, ORP have sometimes been selected based on their clinical skills in the operating theater. To teach on courses, this is not enough. Choosing the right individuals to join AO ORP faculty is complex. Mistakes are expensive in terms of time and money, as well as for credibility of the organization.

■ ▦    **The following suggestions should help you to identify suitable ORP and surgeons both during courses and in practice:**

   ▦ **Has considered reasons for wishing to join faculty.**
   ▦ **Is always well prepared.**
   ▦ **Places a high value on AO principles and philosophy.**
   ▦ **Uses AO techniques in practice.**
   ▦ **Has sincere consideration for work colleagues and learners.**
   ▦ **Listens attentively.**

- **Creates a sense of community among colleagues.**
- **Will be able and willing to contribute to the development of ORP training.**
- **Does not magnify any difficulties in relationships between surgeons and ORP.**
- **Can provide evidence of a commitment to teaching.**

Experience over the last 10 years has shown that a reasonably confident and outgoing personality is also very important.

Steer clear of anyone who:

- Monopolizes conversations or teaching sessions.
- Interrupts constantly.
- Withholds customary social cues such as greetings or head nodding.
- Insults, patronizes, or ridicules anyone.
- Speaks dogmatically, not respecting the opinion of others.
- Complains or whines excessively.
- Criticizes excessively.
- Flatters others insincerely.
- Braggs or shows off.

## 7 Reflection

One major concern is whether an AO course, or indeed any training, makes a difference to practice, and therefore, whether it improves patient care. There is limited evidence to support the universal assumption that training does affect practice. Calderhead [16] observes that many practitioners have implicit or tacit knowledge of principles of practice, but may not have access to it. McLeod et al [17] propose that such tacit knowledge may be acquired and stored in long-term memory, as a consequence of reflection in action, ie, considering the features of an experience as it is happening. Reflection on action, ie, reflection after an experience, may also contribute to the development of tacit knowledge. This activity of reviewing and evaluating often leads to learning and builds expertise [18]. Fortunately, many nurses will already be familiar with the concept of reflective practice from their training. Currently, AO courses are packed with content, leaving little space for such activity. However, ORP faculty members are encouraging reflection at every opportunity, particularly during the discussions, to increase the likelihood of achieving lasting change.

Course participants need to explore explicitly how to make and maintain change to current practice. If they clearly identify the changes they want to make to their practice and how they plan to make them before they leave the course, they are more likely to achieve permanent change. Again, it is essential to provide an opportunity at the end of the course for such planning.

## 8    Conclusion

The similarities between ORP and surgeons' courses are greater than the differences. However, issues concerned with diversity can be magnified on an ORP course, and faculty—particularly surgical faculty—must be sensitive to such issues. Because teachers on ORP courses are from different professional backgrounds, more time and energy is required to develop a cohesive and effective faculty. Whether teaching ORP or surgeons, moving from monocultural/gender/professional communities to highly diverse communities is a worldwide phenomenon, which will become even greater given the increase in mobility and communications [4].

Perhaps the most important attribute of a successful ORP faculty member is their unerring belief that the role of the ORP matters and in which it is worth investing time and effort. Those who struggle to recognize the unique contribution of the ORP, whether surgeon or ORP, would be better placed on uniprofessional courses, where their values and beliefs will not interfere with learning.

■ ⫶    **"Better educated ORP deliver more considered care" [19]. Such optimism, however, depends on widespread acceptance of the importance of the "better educated ORP".**

## 9 Anecdotes

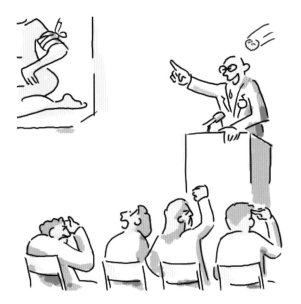

Within the first three slides of a lecture on bone healing, early on in the course, the surgeon lecturer showed a graphic slide of a semi-clad woman in a provocative pose. While he giggled loudly, he failed to notice the lack of response from the audience. Although most appeared to find the image fairly innocuous, nobody laughed and several gave clear signals that they found it offensive. Those who were clearly offended bristled in the audience, affecting those around them. By slide 5 most of the participants had stopped concentrating as they either looked bemused, embarrassed or angry. The member of faculty, who then struggled with his discussion and practical groups, was asked to apologize for his error of judgment, and has not taught on an AO course since.

Having been invited as faculty to an ORP course on the other side of the world, Jo arrived early to spend the day working with ORP staff in the maxillofacial trauma theater. She was able to scrub in on cases to experience surgical practice from an ORP standpoint. She was also able to spend breaks talking to ORP on a more informal basis to find out what issues were the highest priority for them in terms of learning. By the next day Jo had invaluable insight into the culture of surgical and ORP practice and had started to build some relationships with other ORP faculty. Perhaps of even greater importance, participants were aware of Jo's special efforts to prepare for their course, which resulted in establishment of rapport more quickly and effectively.

Lisa Hadfield-Law

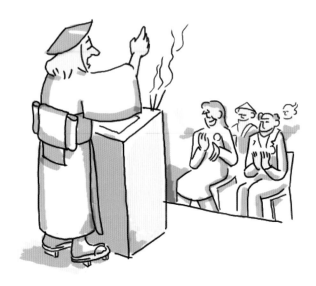

## 10    Bibliography

1. **Rosen J, Spatz ES, Gaaserud AM, et al** (2004) A new approach to developing cross-cultural communication skills. *Med Teach*; 26(2):126–32.
2. **Baldwin D** (1999) Community-based experiences and cultural competence. *Journal of Nursing Education*; 38(5):195–196.
3. **Rogers A** (1986) *Teaching Adults.* Milton Keynes: Open University Press.
4. **Kachur EK, Altshuler L** (2004) Cultural competence is everyone's responsibility! *Med Teach*; 26(2):101–5.
5. **Grantcharov TP, Bardram L, Funch-Jensen P, et al** (2003) Impact of hand dominance, gender, and experience with computer games on performance in virtual reality laparoscopy. *Surg Endosc*; 17(7):1082–5.
6. **Schueneman AL, Pickleman J, Freeark RJ** (1985) Age, gender, lateral dominance, and prediction of operative skill among general surgery residents. *Surgery*; 98(3):506–15.
7. **Hitchcock MA, Stritter FT, Bland CJ** (1993) Faculty development in health professions: conclusions and recommendations. *Medical Teacher*; 14(4):295–319.
8. **Levinson W, Weiner J** (1991) Promotion and tenure of women and minorities on medical school faculties. *Annals of Internal Medicine*; 114:63–68.
9. **Karle H** (2004) International trends in medical education: diversification contra convergence. *Medical Teacher*; 26(3):205–206.
10. **Davies C** (1995) *Gender and the professional predicament in nursing.* Milton Keynes: Open University Press.
11. **Kitson AL** (1996) Does nursing have a future? *BMJ*; 313:1647–1651.
12. **Showers B, Joyce B** (1996) The evolution of peer coaching. *Educational Leadership*; 53(6):12–16.
13. **Joyce B, Showers B** (1982) The coaching of teaching. *Educational Leadership*; 40(1):4–10.
14. **Knowles M** (1990) *The Adult Learner: a neglected species.* 4th ed. Houston: Gulf.
15. **Bellodi PL** (2004) The general practitioner and the surgeon: stereotypes and medical specialties. *Rev Hosp Clin Fac Med SPaulo*; 59(1):15–24.
16. **Calderhead J** (1996) Teachers' beliefs and knowledge. *Berliner DC, Calfee RC, (eds) Handbook of Educational Psychology.* New York: McMillan, 709–729.
17. **McLeod PJ, Meagher T, Steinert Y, et al** (2004) Clinical teachers' tacit knowledge of basic pedagogic principles. *Medical Teacher*; 26(1):23–7.
18. **Schon DA** (1983) *The Reflective Practitioner.* New York: Basic Books.
19. **Miers M.** (2002) Nurse education in higher education. *Nurse Education Today*; 22:212–219.

Authors   Joseph S Green, Piet G de Boer, and David Davis

# 8    Summary and future directions for AO education

The purpose of this final chapter is two-fold—to summarize the major conceptual foundations of the suggestions made in the previous chapters of the book and look forward to the future of AO education by applying the concepts found in the recent literature to the realities of surgeons in the educational roles they play within AO.

## 1    Summary of educational concepts

The focus of this book has been on how to improve the educational practices of AO clinicians as they participate in various educational roles within the organization—course chairman, discussion group leader, practical director, table instructor, lecturer, and ORP faculty member. For each of these chapters the two authors combined their expertise and formulated multiple practical suggestions to assist in carrying out these roles in the most effective and efficient way possible. Their advice was based on real world experience and sound educational principles. In reviewing these suggestions, six overriding concepts emerge:

- Meticulous planning and dealing with details and the unexpected.
- Collaborative linkage of concepts and people.
- Dealing with the differences in the learning environment and the learners that exist in the worldwide AO community.
- Using multiple educational roles and methods to facilitate learning.
- Facilitating learner interaction and application to practice.
- Providing feedback, motivation, and clear expectations of outcomes.

## 1.1 Meticulous planning and dealing with details and the unexpected

The principles that were discussed throughout the book relating to planning include:

- Use a comprehensive process that includes identification of learning needs; setting of objectives; selection of formats, methods, and media; faculty selection; translation of new knowledge into the practice setting; managing resources and time; and evaluation (see 2 How to be a course chairman).
- Be deliberate and well-organized, while managing your time and budget effectively and efficiently (see 2 How to be a course chairman).
- Learn as much as possible from the past to improve the future (see 2 How to be a course chairman and 7 How to run an ORP course).
- Allow sufficient time in your planning to better handle the unexpected (see 2 How to be a course chairman).
- Use the precourse to help everyone prepare well in advance (see 3 How to run a discussion group).
- Stay on time with careful planning and anticipating possible troubles (see 5 How to be a table instructor).
- Rehearse and rehearse and KISS: keeping it short and simple (see 6 How to give a lecture).

## 1.2 Collaborative linkage of concepts and people

These principles, that appeared in many of the chapters, deal with the important educational responsibility of establishing linkages to assure success:

- Collaborate with fellow planners and faculty to assure coordination. Talk with others—don't try to do it all on your own (see 2 How to be a course chairman and 7 How to run an ORP course).
- Select colleagues for educational roles based on their skills and interests (see 2 How to be a course chairman and 7 How to run an ORP course).
- Work with colleague faculty and support staff as one team (see 2 How to be a course chairman). Organize content that clearly links to other content, skills, and past knowledge (see 3 How to run a discussion group).
- Link case studies and cases to previous lectures (see 3 How to run a discussion group).
- Create "learnable chunks" of content to facilitate learning and retention (see 4 How to run a practical).
- Use evidence-based content (see 6 How to give a lecture).
- Provide opportunities for practice of skills discussed (see 6 How to give a lecture).

## 1.3    Dealing with multiple differences in the environment and among learners

Effective education depends on how well those who are doing the planning take into account the myriad differences among those who participate in the AO activities. These differences include:

- Use tracking to account for various skill levels of learners, as well as different learning style preferences that use different senses (see 2 How to be a course chairman and 3 How to run a discussion group).
- Understand that international membership means that language and other cultural differences require strategies to address these, such as simultaneous translation or multiple meetings (see 3 How to run a discussion group, 5 How to be a table instructor, and 7 How to run an ORP course).
- Prepare the learning environment in advance to account for possible problems and various adjustments that might need to be made to increase the effectiveness of the education (see 3 How to run a discussion group).
- Match the targeted level of the information to be provided with the current level of knowledge of the learners and their legitimate expectations to prevent "missing" the target audience (see 6 How to give a lecture and 7 How to run an ORP course).
- Use supplemental information such as handouts to support learning (see 6 How to give a lecture).

## 1.4    Using multiple educational roles and methods to facilitate learning

Being responsive to learners requires flexibility in dealing with the planning and implementation of the activities. Those concepts that are specifically mentioned throughout the book include:

- Use focused group discussions, cases, and evidence (see 3 How to run a discussion group).
- Match appropriate methods with certain objectives or content and make sure lectures and videos are mutually supportive (see 4 How to run a practical).
- Learn how to serve multiple roles such as coach, mentor, and facilitator (see 5 How to be a table instructor and 7 How to run an ORP course).

## 1.5    Facilitating learner interaction and application to practice

There are many suggestions made in several chapters, including:

- Involve learners in their own learning activities by increasing interactivity (see 2 How to be a course chairman and 5 How to be a table instructor).
- Develop a creative atmosphere in the learning environment that facilitates discussion and mutual respect (see 3 How to run a discussion group and 7 How to run an ORP course).
- Keep groups small, to 6–8 people, when discussion is desired (see 3 How to run a discussion group).
- Use ARS in larger sessions to give participants multiple opportunities to interact with faculty, the content, and fellow learners (see 3 How to run a discussion group and 6 How to give a lecture).

- Give learners the chance to integrate their experience with the content of their learning (see 5 How to be a table instructor and 7 How to run an ORP course).
- Facilitate learners meeting each other (see 5 How to be a table instructor).

### 1.6 Providing feedback, motivation, and clear expectations of outcomes

This final category of concepts involves helping learners, faculty, and other planners by focusing on some of the motivators and results of participation in AO courses:

- Start the planning and the implementation of actual activities with clearly stated expectations for outcomes based on what was learned from past courses (see 2 How to be a course chairman and 6 How to give a lecture).
- Focus on the expectation that learners will use the information and skills taught to them to increase the quality of the care they provide patients (see 2 How to be a course chairman, 5 How to be a table instructor, and 7 How to run an ORP course).
- Let learners know what they don't know through the use of pretests, cases, discussions, or ARS as valuable feedback that increases motivation to learn (see 2 How to be a course chairman, 3 How to run a practical, and 5 How to be a table instructor).
- Determine learners' readiness to change to make necessary enhancements to the learning processes (see 2 How to be a course chairman and 6 How to give a lecture).

- Provide reinforcement of learning after the formal activity (see 3 How to run a discussion group).
- Help learners apply theories that have been taught to their actual practice of skills during learning and back in the practice setting (see 3 How to run a discussion group, 4 How to run a practical, 5 How to be a table instructor, and 7 How to run an ORP course).
- Evaluate all aspects of the educational planning and implementation process (see 2 How to be a course chairman, 3 How to run a discussion group, 4 How to run a practical, 5 How to be a table instructor, and 6 How to give a lecture).
- Explain, demonstrate, involve, coach, and test— EDICT (see 4 How to run a practical).
- Use "advance organizers" before starting activities and summarize as you progress into the activity (see 4 How to run a practical).
- Provide emotional support to learners, planners, staff, and faculty to facilitate learning (see 5 How to be a table instructor and 7 How to run an ORP course).
- Help learners understand their areas of discrepancy between what is and what ought to be (see 5 How to be a table instructor).

## 2    Future trends in education

Clinicians and educators experienced in the continuing professional development of physicians postulate that many forces for change will direct developments in CME over the next decade. These are important trends for the medical profession as a whole, but will have an impact on the discipline of orthopedic surgery in distinct and important ways. Five future trends have been identified:

- **Self-assessment programs (SAP).**
- **Problem-based learning (PBL).**
- **Continuous quality improvement (CQI).**
- **Educational technologies (ET).**
- **Knowledge management (KM).**

To at least some extent, these five domains overlap. SAP, PBL, and CQI have mutual interdependencies and represent a continuum of sorts—self-assessment requiring the use of internal, subjective and reflective skills, and CQI utilizing more external, practice-based and objective sources. Further, "knowledge management", the ability to detect needs for knowledge and to understand how and where to find it, the skills to critically appraise the evidence and those which enable the surgeon to subsequently (and appropriately) apply the new information drawn from each of the SAP, PBL, and CQI. Finally, somewhat orthogonal to each of these areas, yet of true interest to all, is the advent and increasing utilization of education and quality improvement technologies.

In each of these five areas, several papers have been selected by means of a focused literature search, using the Research & Development Resource Base in Continuing Education (RDRB available at http://www.cme.utoronto.ca/search), operated by the Knowledge Translation Program of the Faculty of Medicine, University of Toronto. Using the keywords captured above in each of these areas, articles from the 14,000-item database were extracted, reviewed by the authors for their currency and their representation of future trends. They were subsequently systematically reviewed and are summarized below.

### 2.1    Self-assessment programs

Self-assessment is defined as the ability to reflect on one's performance or competencies, and to respond to this assessment by developing learning objectives to meet defined educational needs or clinical performance gaps. In general, these competencies may be subdivided into knowledge, skills, and attitudes. Several major articles demonstrate the ways in which self-assessment may evolve in the ensuring years.

MacDonald and colleagues [1] outline the standard measures of self-assessment of knowledge in the surgical disciplines. Identifying major issues beyond the assessment of knowledge, Parboosingh and his colleagues [2] have articulated key challenges facing the future of competency assessment. These are of particular importance in the surgical specialties and include the assessment of surgical skills, the determination of ongoing competence, and the appropriate acquisition of new skills. Further challenges include the abilities:

- **To ensure reliability and validity, level of assessment appropriate to the clinical practices, and scope of the physician.**
- **To determine the life-long and self-directed learning skills of clinicians.**
- **To create assessment tools in the realm of ethics and professionalism.**

Lockyer et al [3] outlined a "360-degree assessment process", adapting this method from the business and organizational literature. This model differs from others in that it reflects a further trend—that of governments, regulatory bodies, health care systems, hospitals, and others—to weigh in on the assessment process, adding an objective assurance of competence. The 360-degree model uses a carefully selected steering committee that chooses appropriate professionals who have first hand knowledge of the individual's performance, develops questionnaires and other measures to evaluate that performance, and sets the standards for ethical and reliable measures. According to the author, however, feedback gained from this process, used to guide physician performance, appears to be relatively ineffective in changing surgical behavior—a subject of further study.

### Implications for AO
AO faculty will all be more involved in self-assessment processes over the next few years.

■ ▪ **One of the valuable services that could be provided by AO would be systematic self-assessment tools based on the critical skills being taught in AO courses.**

The data could be used as needs assessment for the courses and to assist faculty in dividing their learners into more homogenous groups for more effective and efficient learning. The data might also be used by the participants to begin gathering information on their own surgical competencies for use in their hospital and private practice.

Self-assessment tools have been used by AO for many years. Distance learning material (DLM) has been available for the AO Principles Course for the past decade in printed form. This material includes test-retest material, but has not met with good acceptance from the course participants.

Self-assessment material was successfully used in the 2003 pelvis and acetabular course in Bad Homburg, where it was used to select two groups from within the course participants—experienced and novice. This exercise allowed the course to be structured in such a way to assure that the educational needs of each group were fully met.

Self-assessment cases have been available on the AO website for the past 2 years for the use by course participants who had attended AO courses in Davos. This material has proven to be very popular with the course participants, even though generating this material is extremely time consuming. The development of the AO portal will further increase the number of cases that can be used for self-assessment.

### 2.2 Problem-based learning

PBL may be defined as learning by discussing and interacting with case or patient materials–either simulated or real. Many methods for PBL exist from simple case discussions prompted by paper or presented cases, the use of standardized patients, or complicated surgical simulations. (These last are discussed in 8 Summary and future directions for AO education; 2.4 Educational technologies.)

Is PBL effective? A relatively recent review of several randomized controlled trials of small group, tutor-led problem-based formats [4] sheds only some light on the question of the effect of PBL on satisfaction of learning, the competencies and physician performance change or health care outcomes. The picture is mixed. Based on cautious support from the literature in undergraduate medical education, the authors found only six studies of PBL methods in relatively well-designed studies. Of these, the authors conclude that there is only limited evidence about the effect of these methods on physician knowledge or performance, and only moderate evidence that physicians were more satisfied with their learning than with traditional methods. Painted against this rather cautious background, another article [5] describes studies using small group (5–10 participants) and larger group (10–40) PBL sessions in CME. Though less rigorous methodologically than those studies referenced by Smits, this trial's results indicate a more optimistic view of the format—participants perceived the PBL program to be more effective than those which were lecture based and changed their performance as measured by prescribing rates and utilization of urgent care.

### Implications for AO
The use of problem-based case studies is integral to the success of AO courses.

■ ▪  **Perhaps the AO should begin some research as to the relative effectiveness of the use of these educational methods as compared to other small group methods that involve learners more in their own learning.**

Problem-based learning has been an integral part of spinal education for many years. The interactive spine course is held in Davos and is based entirely around discussions concerning real clinical problems.

The videos used in AO practicals are also being revised to bring in clinically relevant information. Course participants often find it difficult to relate the plastic bone model exercise to clinical cases. The new video format will try to relate each exercise to a clinical case. The new format will also include material taken from surgery to better increase the participants' understanding of the exercise.

Core material also exists for the principles and advances course discussion groups. This material consists of clinical cases with relevant information as well as x-rays. The group discussion leader is also provided with details of the learning objectives of each case presentation.

Interactive problem-based case studies are also now available on the AO portal. All course participants in Davos will have access to this material.

### 2.3    Continuous quality improvement

The aims of CQI are clearly imbedded in its name—increasing the quality of care delivered to patients on a regular basis. This is clearly a natural goal for health care practitioners. CQI, however, unlike PBL and SAP, speaks to the need to improve systems of care, recognizing that there are many factors (eg, operating room policies, training of OR nurses, and availability of resources).

Much of the impetus for this movement in health care has come from the Institute of Medicine's report, "Crossing the Quality Chasm", which states, "health care today harms too frequently and routinely fails to deliver its potential benefits" [6]. Perhaps the most persuasive and articulate of authors in the field of CQI, Berwick [7], calls for all clinicians and their colleagues in the health care system to set clear health care improvement targets, monitor progress, and change the way the work is done to reach the goals. Although this work is less recent than others quoted in this chapter, this articulation of the movement in CQI is seminal and will have profound effects on medical practice in the decades to come.

■ ▪ **Among many grand aims Berwick [7] articulated are those with possible impact on the surgical disciplines. They include a call for reduction in inappropriate surgeries, treating underlying causes of illness and trauma (eg, encouraging helmet use for bike riders) and unnecessary end-of-life care procedures and treatments unwanted by the patient.**

An excellent example of CQI methods in the area of surgery is described by Ferguson et al [8]. In a randomized controlled trial, the authors used CQI methods to improve process measures in coronary artery bypass graft surgery. Similarly, Brown et al [9] describe a similar approach to guideline implementation in pediatric surgery.

Finally, demonstrating that the CQI approach is permanent, Moore and Pennington [10] describe practice-based learning and improvement (PBLI) as a "collection of activities that (clinicians) engage in to link opportu-nities for improvement with resources that can address those opportunities". They note the increasing pressures for health systems to improve care and change physician behavior. They also point out the wide variations in practice and the lack of effect of traditional continuing education as prime movers behind the PBLI and CQI movements.

**Implications for AO**

Perhaps AO might develop tools that the participants can use to measure and improve their own surgical skills in their practice setting or AO activities might require participants to bring this type of data with them to an AO course for individual or small group discussions on how to improve performance. Evaluation of skills is extremely complex, time consuming, and expensive. There is also the concern in many regions of the world that AO should not be acting as an examining board.

■ ▪ **The newly implemented AO course evaluation process is beginning to focus on how the participants are able to use the information provided in AO courses to improve their practice (see 1 AO education—introduction).**

**2.4 Educational technologies**

Ho et al [11] describe a process they call TEKT, or technology-enabled knowledge translation, implying the use of a wide variety of technical aids to assist the practitioner or the health care system in acquiring knowledge and applying it in an appropriate manner. This excellent overview article provides a framework for understanding the nature of technology-enabled knowledge transfer, offers a discussion of the issues involved in implementing such systems and establishes an evaluation framework to assess its success.

- Simulation technology for training and assessment: There are many forces that lead to the use of simulation technologies for skills training and for assessment purposes. Issenberg and his colleagues [12] describe these forces as changes in health care that limit time and that reduce the availability of patient resources for training, and expanding options for diagnosis, and management by the new technologies themselves. This article refers to four areas of high technology use: laparoscopic techniques, cardiovascular disease simulators, anesthesia simulators, and finally multimedia computer systems that create and use case-based programs.

  ■    **There is evidence that using simulations as "virtual reality training" leads to quicker adoption of laparoscopic techniques on the part of surgeons [13].**

  Simulations can enable team training in resuscitation [14], enables the teaching of emergency response skills in the military [15], and that (at least in trainees) improvements in self-assessment of performance and accuracy of error estimation [1]. Clearly some surgical procedures lend themselves more easily to virtual reality procedure. Arthroscopic and laparoscopic techniques are particularly suitable for this form of teaching. We are, however, a long way from the technologies that allow the assessment of a pilot's skill using a simulator. The development of computer technology may allow in the future the development of useful surgical reality training. But this is probably at least a decade away.

- Communication technology:

  ■    **New technologies exist in the area of computerized information sharing both of the more transitional, desktop type, and of the personal digital assistant or "handheld".**

  PDAs convey information, often in abbreviated fashion, at the point of care—the office, surgical suite, bedside, emergency room, or in other care settings. As Sinkov et al [16] say, "The Internet…is becoming a more integral part of orthopedic education every day". Their article on the specific subject of online orthopedic surgery CME accomplishes three tasks: it reviews many orthopedic web-based resources (eg, websites: Orthogate, OrthoNet, AO North America, American Academy of Orthopedic Surgery, South Australian Orthopedic Registrar), it surveys the use of online resources by trainees and practicing orthopedic surgeons, and it lays out a plan for a comprehensive, constantly updated orthopedic online resource. The gap in Internet use between surgeons in training (100%) and those who are practicing (79%) is not surprising, but does point to increased use of these resources in the future. Lugo-Vicente [17], in a similar review of Internet-based resources for surgeons, describes adjuncts to this learning medium including electronic mail, discussion groups, file transfer, and list-serves. One further article on the use of the Internet [18] points out the global ramifications for international health; here surgeons can develop skills online, consult with experts, learn new information, all at remote, international sites.

- Distance education technology:
  The use of distance education techniques such as web- and video-casting, are methods by which teachers communicate new diagnostic methods, surgical procedures, pre- and postoperative management and other clinical issues to their learners.

**Implications for AO**

■ ▥ **The development of the AO portal is an important step in the application of communication technology within the AO.**

The portal will offer surgical modules in which the user can identify the clinical problem, which he is faced with in practice, and receive advice as to possible solutions. These surgical modules are based around anatomical regions of the body. The user is offered a set of x-rays and can choose which x-rays best match those of his patient. The user is then led through an algorithm which will in the end inform him of the possible clinical options together with their advantages and disadvantages. The surgical modules on the AO portal will be available in July 2005.

### 2.5   Knowledge management

■ ▥ **Knowledge management is a complex phenomenon in a highly complex clinical world, marked by information overload.**

These issues attending KM are also multifactorial, ranging—as seen from the selection of articles in this area—from those related to the clinician to those related to the health system within which they practice.

- Clinician issues:
  Dawes and Sampson, in a recent review of physicians' information seeking behaviors [19] describe the results of 19 studies, using questionnaires, interviews, and observation. They confirm that print materials and talking to colleagues form the backbone of information gathering on the part of clinicians. This finding has not changed in the last 20 years. They note, however, several barriers to information-gathering including accessibility, timeliness, and format; these are clearly areas which—with increasingly sophisticated search computerized knowledge management mechanisms—technology can provide an answer.

- System issues:
  Parboosingh describes one of the current "hot concepts" in CME, that of "communities of practice" (COPs)—groups of clinicians who share an interest in a clinical area and who engage in collective learning which creates bonds between and among them. Like journal clubs, but with a heavier emphasis on shared learning and experience, these COPs can more readily deal with information retrieval, critique, synthesis, and management than individual physicians [20].

**Implications for AO**

■ ▥ **In a very real sense AO is a community of practice. It is a group of clinicians sharing an interest and working together.**

AO members may treat patients in a variety of ways, but their practice is based on a common philosophy. Community members may disagree about the way in which an individual patient is treated but they hold a common belief that their purpose is to improve the care of patients.

## 3    Bibliography

With acknowledgement to Laure Perrier, MLS, MEd, Information Specialist, and Joanne Goldman, MA, Research Associate, Knowledge Transation Program, Faculty of Medicine, University of Toronto, for collecting and summarizing the literature.

1. **MacDonald J, Williams RG, Rogers DA** (2000) Self-assessment in simulation-based surgical skills training. *Am J Surg*; 185(4):319–322.

2. **Parboosingh J** (2000) Credentialing physicians: Challenges for continuing medical education. *J Contin Educ Health Prof*; 20(3):188–190.

3. **Lockyer J** (2003) Multisource Feedback in the Assessment of Physician Competencies. *JCEHP*; 23(1):4.

4. **Smits PB, Verbeek JH, de Buisonje CD** (2002) Problem based learning in continuing medical education: A review of controlled evaluation studies. *BMJ*; 324(7330):153–156.

5. **Zeitz HJ** (1999) Problem based learning: Development of a new strategy for effective continuing medical education. *Allergy Asthma Proc*; 20(5):317–321.

6. **Institute of Medicine** (2001). Crossing the quality chasm: A new health system for the 21st century/ Committee on Quality Health Care in America, Institute of Medicine. Washington, DC: National Academy Press.

7. **Berwick DM** (1994) Eleven worthy aims for clinical leadership of health system reform. *JAMA*; 272:797–802.

8. **Ferguson TB, Jr, Peterson ED, Coombs LP, et al** (2003) Use of continuous quality improvement to increase use of process measures in patients undergoing coronary artery bypass graft surgery: A randomized controlled trial. *JAMA*; 290(1):49–56.

9. **Brown JJ, Wacogne I, Fleckney S, et al** (2004) Achieving early surgery for undescended testes: quality improvement through a multifaceted approach to guideline implementation. *Child Care Health Dev*; 30(2):97–102.

10. **Moore DE, Jr, Pennington FC** (2003) Practice-based learning and improvement. *J Contin Educ Health Prof*; 23(suppl 1):S73–S80.

11. **Ho K, Bloch R, Gondocz T, et al** (2004) Technology-enabled knowledge translation: Frameworks to promote research and practice. *J Contin Educ Health Prof*; 24(2):90–99.

12. **Issenberg SB, McGaghie WC, Hart IR, et al** (1999) Simulation technology for healthcare professional skills training and assessment. *JAMA*; 282(9):861–866.

13. **Jordan JA, Gallagher AG, McGuigan J, et al** (2001) Virtual reality training leads to faster adaptation to the novel psychomotor restrictions encountered by laparoscopic surgeons. *Surg Endosc*; 15(10):1080–1084.

14. **Holcomb JB, Dumire RD, Crommett JW, et al** (2002) Evaluation of trauma team performance using an advanced human patient simulator for resuscitation training. *J Trauma*; 52(6):1078–1085.

15. **Freeman KM, Thompson SF, Allely EB, et al** (2001) A virtual reality patient simulation system for teaching emergency response skills to U.S. Navy medical providers. *Prehospital Disaster Med*; 16(1):3–8.

16. **Sinkov VA, Andres BM, Wheeless CR, et al** (2004) Internet-based learning. *Clin Orthop*; Apr(421):99–106.

17. **Lugo-Vicente H** (2000) Internet resources and web pages for pediatric surgeons. *Semin Pediatr Surg*; 9(1):11–18.

18. **Zbar RI, Otake LR, Miller MJ, et al** (2001) Web-based medicine as a means to establish centers of surgical excellence in the developing world. *Plast Reconstr Surg*; 108(2):460–465.

19. **Dawes M, Sampson U** (2003) Knowledge management in clinical practice: a systematic review of information seeking behavior in physicians. *Int J Med Inf*. 2003; 71(1):9–15.

20. **Parboosingh JT** (2002) Physician communities of practice: Where learning and practice are inseparable. *J Contin Educ Health Prof*; 22(4):230–236.

# Appendix—AO courses using cadaveric material

## Guidelines

The AO Education Steering Board set up certain guidelines for courses using cadaveric material. It is the course chairman's responsibility to validate the venue as suitable to hold such a course as well as to ensure that the regulations will be followed as outlined in the document. Only upon written confirmation to the AO can such a course be accepted and material provided for practical exercises.

Each course participant—prior to commencing the course—must sign a waiver of liability (see sample) and it is the course chairman's responsibility that the original copy is retained for submission to AO International. The original forms will be archived should any legal issues arise at a later date.

## Regulations

The use of cadaveric material during AO courses improves teaching in certain aspects. The potential for infection both to course participants and those handling the instrumentation is such that the AO Foundation and the industrial partner have defined regulations that must be followed for each course. These regulations are mandatory for all persons organizing cadaver courses. No such course will be approved by the AO if the following regulations are not adhered to.

1. Courses using cadaveric material may only be conducted in accordance with the following prerequisites.
2. Courses must be conducted in an approved institution designed for anatomical teaching purposes.
3. All cadaveric material used must carry a certificate of bacteriological and virological sterility given by the institution providing the cadaveric material.
4. Only prepared cadavers should be used on AO courses. No fresh cadaveric material is to be used unless the above certification is guaranteed.
5. All instruments used for cadaver courses should be kept apart from other course material.
6. All course material (excluding implants) that is to be shipped back to the industrial partner must be subject to a decontamination* and cleaning* procedure before trans-shipment.
7. All material used in cadaver courses will be subjected to full hospital sterilization carried out by the producer on return of the instruments.
8. Course organizers are responsible for providing, decontaminating, cleaning, and sterilizing the general instruments used for surgical approaches.
9. All implants used should be single use only. No implants used in cadaver specimens may be trans-shipped back to the industrial partner.
   (If the course organizers choose to reuse the implants for further courses with cadavers, they do so at their own risk. They are responsible for the decontamination, cleaning, and sterilizing of these implants.)
10. The costs of the implants must be covered by the course fees and will be invoiced at a special price.
11. Course organizers must make available gloves, gowns, and masks to all course participants and technical staff. Safety glasses or goggles should also be made available where there is a risk of aerosols or droplet spread, for example, drilling.
12. Exercises with dry bones are to be conducted in a separate room using separate material.
13. This regulation sheet must be signed by the course chairman and returned to AO International before the course will be approved.
14. The liability waiver form (attached) must be signed by each registered participant prior to commencing the course.

* According to local standards and requirements for hospital instrument decontamination and cleaning.

## AO courses with cadaver specimens—waiver of liability

The undersigned fully acknowledges the following:

- His/her attendance and participation in this educational course under the auspices of the AO Foundation ("AO educational course") will involve contact with cadaver specimens.
- The cadaver specimens will be prepared and certified disease-free by a third party company fully independent of the AO Foundation.
- Even with such certification, the total absence of any kind of pathogenic organism cannot be guaranteed by the AO Foundation.

In consideration of this, the undersigned for himself, his personal representatives, heirs and next of kin, hereby releases the AO Foundation, its directors, officers, employees representatives, or any natural or legal person related to or in connection with the AO Foundation of any and all liability to the undersigned, his personal representatives, heirs and next of kin, for any injury, disease or any other loss or damage that may occur during or after the AO educational course or caused directly or indirectly by the attendance and participation of the undersigned in the AO educational course.

I have read, understood, and I fully agree with the above.

Name/first name:

Signature:

Date:

Course and date:

Location:

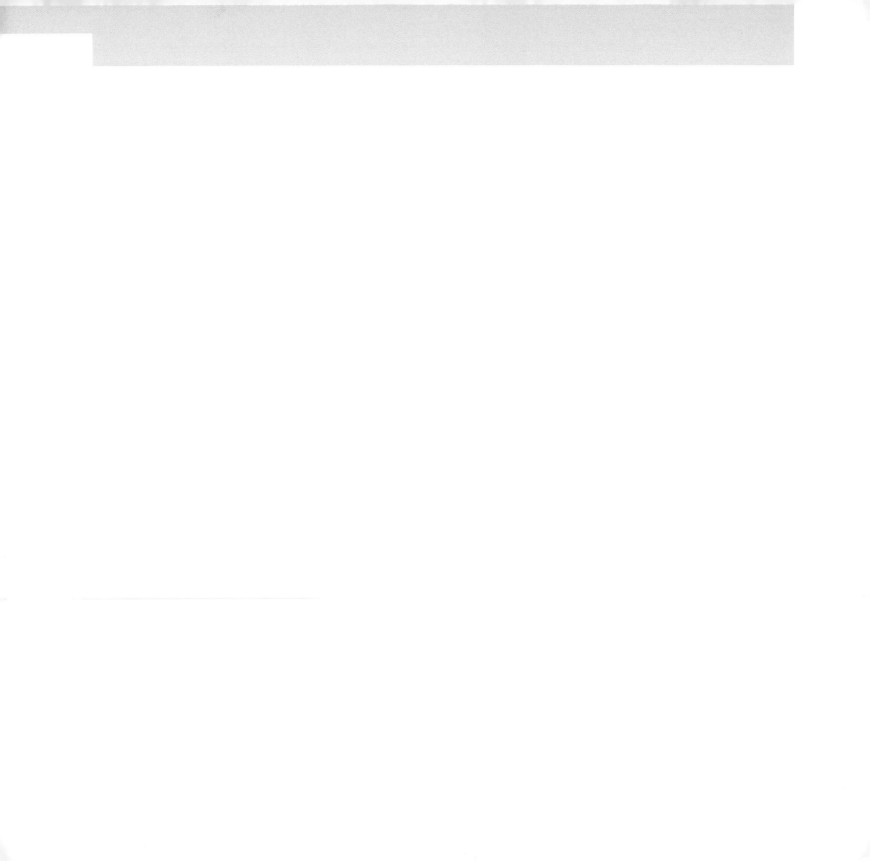